I0797888

Praise for *Liberating Yoga*

"A beautifully articulated and deeply insightful work by Harpinder, enriched with wisdom drawn from her life experiences. The book is both engaging and relatable, sure to inspire readers on their own journey of transformation."

—Sri Prasad Rangnekar, founder of Yogaprasad Institute

"Honest, raw, and straightforward. In *Liberating Yoga*, Harpinder Kaur Mann motivates the sincere practitioner of yoga to look beyond the conventional lens and take their yoga Journey forward by leaning into its roots, culture, and philosophy. She made a convincing point why context in yoga matters more than sterile and robotic techniques. Be ready to leave inspired, stirred, yet stilled."

—Indu Arora, author of *SOMA: 100 Heritage Recipes for Self-Care, YOGA: Ancient Heritage Tomorrow's Vision*, and *MUDRA: The Sacred Secret*

"*Liberating Yoga* is a bold, necessary offering for all who care about the integrity of yoga. Harpinder Kaur Mann weaves her intimate knowledge of yoga, Sikh heritage and personal journey with a deep respect for yoga's roots, reminding us that yoga is not just a practice—it's a path of connection, liberation, and healing. In a world where yoga has been commodified, she beautifully reclaims its authentic essence, showing us how to honor both its cultural and spiritual heritage with compassion and respect. This book is an essential read for those who wish to engage with yoga responsibly, while embracing its true purpose."

—Susanna Barkataki, author of *Ignite Your Yoga* and *Embrace Yoga's Roots*

"*Liberating Yoga* exposes how the West has exploited yoga's sacred tree of knowledge, extracting only the limbs of postures and breathwork from its rich cultural soil, while ignoring the deep roots of ethics and wisdom that bear its medicinal fruit of liberation. Harpinder Kaur Mann emerges as a confident voice of a new generation of trauma-informed yoga activists, skillfully calling us in to face the shadow of the colonial mindset—not only to restore the integrity of the yoga tradition, but to allow it to heal the very source of our fragmented psyche and fractured society. This is timely medicine."

—Dr. Miles Neale, PsyD, Buddhist psychotherapist and author of *Gradual Awakening* and *Return with Elixir*

"In *Liberating Yoga*, Harpinder offers insights, guidance, and clarity to trace a path to yoga free of modern day white-washed commercialization. From personal experience, the wisdom of those who came before, and the illuminating truths of the practice, Harpinder lovingly calls on every single reader to join the cause of redirecting yoga from a gimmicky fitness exercise to a holistic, contemplative discipline."

—Tejal Patel, organizer of Tejal Yoga & abcdyogi, co-creator of Yoga is Dead

"Harpinder's pure heart and sense of devotion are evident in this honest telling of her spiritual journey. The reader is treated to a story written with such sincerity and generosity of spirit that you cannot help but read more. I am grateful this story is being shared with the world."

—Reggie Hubbard, founder and Chief Serving Officer, Active Peace LLC; Activist, Strategist and Teacher

"*Liberating Yoga* by Harpinder Kaur Mann is a deeply personal and thought-provoking exploration of yoga as a path to healing, self-acceptance, and cultural reclamation. What sets this book apart is its honest examination of modern yoga, which often exclude marginalized voices and overlook the full spectrum of yoga. Her writing invites readers to reimagine yoga beyond exercise, positioning it as a tool for personal and collective liberation. Harpinder's reflections encourage all of us to embrace our whole selves and engage in the practice of yoga as an act of inner transformation, community healing, and reconnection with ancestral wisdom. Whether you are a long-time practitioner or someone looking for more depth in your practice, *Liberating Yoga* is a timely and inspiring read."

—Manoj Dias, meditation teacher; author of *Still Together*

"*Liberating Yoga* is an absolute joy. Mann's remarkable work sheds light on an ongoing and significant issue in the yoga industry: the appropriation of yoga culture and the creation of an exclusive practice that lacks adaptability and historical understanding. This book is an excellent resource for exploring how yoga can serve as a powerful tool for collective healing and care."

—Dianne Bondy, RYT, Equity Advocate,
and author of *Yoga for Everyone*

"Right from the introduction of *Liberating Yoga* Harpinder Kaur Mann poetically reflects on what many of us who have chosen to practice yoga have experienced at some level- the paradox of how we relate to the modern phenomenon of translating yoga practice in the modern West. As a daughter of Indian immigrants, Harpinder gently and very personally calls all of us into contemplating how we can reconcile the split that exists between the cultural roots and traditional aims of yoga practice with the western commodification and cultural appropriation that so often obscures or distorts this vast tradition. She invites all of us who love yoga into an integrity and humility that opens new potentials of healing and belonging."

—Dr. Scott Blossom, founder of Doctor Blossom, Health
Educator, and licensed practitioner of Traditional
Chinese Medicine and integrative Ayurveda

"It's one thing to research and write about liberation, it's another thing to embody it and vulnerably share it with the world. Harpinder is the perfect lighthouse for the message of *Liberating Yoga* during a very tumultuous time where we need yoga the most."

—Indy Rishi Singh, executive director, Cultivating Self

"With poise and clarity, Harpinder reveals how the yoga industry has both failed to take into account populations too often excluded from the banner of mainstream enlightenment and failed to consider the issues that impact South Asian practitioners. Throughout, she thoughtfully and deliberately takes mainstream yoga to task. Still, it is also an invitation. For every case in which she highlights problematic practices, she offers guidance on how to do better. My wish is for every non-South Asian who calls themselves a yoga practitioner (as I do) will read this book in a state of hushed and humble respect."

—Charlotte Nguyen, activist, Buddhist teacher, and Founder of Get Free!

"Honest, revolutionary and brave . . . this book should be required reading for anyone practicing and teaching yoga. This book is a gift and shows us how we can be in right relationship with the practice of yoga."

—Jonelle Lewis, Fitness + Yoga & Meditation Trainer, co-owner of Empowered Yoga Studio, co-founder of Radical Darshan Yoga School

"With every page, you can feel Harpinder's care and reverence for yoga. This book is a gentle yet powerful call to return to yoga's true essence—a gift for all who seek to practice with authenticity and love."

—Zahabiyah Yamasaki, MEd, RYT, trauma-informed educator and consultant and author of *Trauma-Informed Yoga for Survivors of Sexual Assault: Practices for Healing and Teaching with Compassion*

"Harpinder Kaur Mann writes with humility and grace, sharing complex topics on marginalization with great skill. She draws the reader in: her story is also my story. As a 1.5 generation Indian American, yoga therapist, and Ayurvedic doctor, I resonate with Harpinder's calling in of yoga as an inclusive, life-affirming, home-coming, transformative practice. I hear her stories of how Western yoga has commodified Indian cultures, and I appreciate her skillfulness in weaving narrative with theory to help us move forward with more love and liberation collectively. Thank you, Harpinder, for your magnificent contribution. May we heal legacies of generational and cultural trauma in our selves and our communities. Lokah Samastah Sukhino Bhavantu (May all beings in all the worlds be liberated)."

—Vinita Prachi Murarka, Ayurvedic doctor, author, visionary

Liberating Yoga

Liberating YOGA

From Appropriation to Healing

Harpinder Kaur Mann

Broadleaf Books
Minneapolis

LIBERATING YOGA
From Appropriation to Healing

Library of Congress Cataloging-in-Publication Data

Names: Mann, Harpinder Kaur, author.
Title: Liberating yoga : from appropriation to healing / Harpinder Kaur Mann.
Description: Minneapolis : Broadleaf Books, [2024] | Includes bibliographical references.
Identifiers: LCCN 2023058894 (print) | LCCN 2023058895 (ebook) | ISBN 9781506495026 (print) | ISBN 9781506495934 (eBook)
Subjects: LCSH: Yoga--Philosophy. | Imperialism--Psychological aspects. | Spirituality. | Healing.
Classification: LCC B132.Y6 .K358 2024 (print) | LCC B132.Y6 (ebook) | DDC 181/.45--dc23/eng/20240312
LC record available at https://lccn.loc.gov/2023058894
LC ebook record available at https://lccn.loc.gov/2023058895

Cover image: Vecteezy.com
Cover design: Broadleaf Books

Print ISBN: 978-1-5064-9502-6
eBook ISBN: 978-1-5064-9593-4

Printed in India.

CONTENTS

AUTHOR'S NOTE

All students, clients, and interviewees mentioned by name in this book have provided their consent to be included. In cases where individuals preferred to remain anonymous, names and certain identifying details have been changed to protect their privacy. While adjustments have been made to safeguard confidentiality, every effort has been taken to preserve the authenticity and integrity of all of the stories.

Transliteration

To maintain linguistic precision and authenticity, I have used diacritical marks when quoting directly from texts like the Śrī Guru Granth Sāhib Jī and The Yoga Sūtras of Patañjali, helping to convey sounds unique to Gurmukhi and Sanskrit. For other Hindi, Gurmukhi, Pali, Punjabi, and Sanskrit words that are utilized throughout the book, I have used simplified English transliterations for ease of reading. This approach, though imperfect, aims to balance accessibility with respect for linguistic nuances.

For instance, diacritical marks in quotes help distinguish between sounds such as ṣ and ś (both often rendered as "sh" in English) and preserve nasalized sounds like ṇ, ṅ, and ñ, rather than generalizing them as "n." Macrons denote long vowels, as in ā, while short vowels, such as a, remain unmarked. Retroflex consonants (e.g., ṭ) are also retained in the quotes to differentiate them from dental consonants (e.g., t).

Here is a pronunciation guide to provide approximate Sanskrit to English sound equivalents. They are *not* exact equivalents.

Vowels

a	as in "but" (short)
ā	as in "tar" (held twice as long as short a)
i	as in "sit" (short)
ī	as in "seek" (long)
u	as in "push" (short)
ū	as in "fool" (long)
e	as in "they" (always long)
o	as in "go" (always long)
ṛ	as in "cringe"
ṝ	as in "reed"
ḷ	as in "jewelry"
ai	as in "aisle"
au	as in "cow"
ṃ	as in "yum"
ḥ	pronounced as an echo of the preceding vowel; such as "aha" for aḥ

Consonants

k	as in "pick"
kh	as in "blockhead"
g	as in "gate"
gh	as in "ghastly"
ṅ	as in "sing"
c	as in "chap"
ch	as in "staunch"
j	as in "jog"
jh	as in "hedgehog"
ñ	as in "onion"
ṭ	as in "tub"
ṭh	as in "table"
ḍ	as in "dove"

ḍh	as in "redhead"
ṇ	as in "gentle"
t	as in "tea"
th	as in "boathouse"
d	as in "dove"
dh	as in "bloodhound"
n	as in "no"
p	as in "pie"
ph	as in "uphill"
b	as in "butter"
bh	as in "abhor"
m	as in "mum"
y	as in "yellow"
r	as in "rule"
l	as in "love"
v	as in "vine"
ś	as in "shawl"
ṣ	as in "shove"
s	as in "soul"
h	as in "hope"

Note: Retroflex sounds (ṭ, ṭh, ḍ, ḍh, ṇ) are pronounced with the tongue curled back slightly.

Here are some pronunciation examples that show Sanskrit words with the diacritical marks *and* the English transliteration:

Āsana (आसन): Pronounced "aah-sah-nah" and commonly written as Asana; refers to a yoga posture or seat.

Jnāna (ज्ञान): Pronounced "gyah-nah or jya-nah" and commonly written as Jnana; means knowledge.

Puruṣa (पुरुष): Pronounced "poo-roo-shah" and commonly seen written as Purusha; refers to the innermost conscious self or soul in yoga philosophy.

Śakti (शक्ति): Pronounced "shuk-tee" and commonly written as Shakti; means power and is associated with the Goddess or the feminine power of a male divinity.

INTRODUCTION

The Journey to Wholeness

I HAVE SPENT much of my life yearning to feel like I belong. Perhaps, dear one, you have too? This is an innate human characteristic. It is my belief and lived experience that having the philosophy, practices, and connection of yoga is the healing salve many of us are looking for.

Studying yoga in India and reconnecting to my ancestral practices saved my life. Before finding this path, I was riddled with anxiety—wondering how I would ever earn enough money to pay off my credit card debt and student loans, plagued with worry that I was going to be fired from my job for not being "good enough," and partying and drinking too much. I needed to distract myself from the ever-lingering feeling that something was missing from my life and to numb myself from the pain and sadness of feeling disconnected. I was stuck in this cycle of working, drinking in the evening to relax, waking up hungover and anxious—and starting all over again.

This disconnect in me was repaired through yoga. Its practices and tools showed me I didn't need to change myself to be considered worthy or lovable. That I already am lovable, just as I am. Yoga gave me a guidebook to make sense of life. Yoga also taught me that, at times, I will be lost and clueless—and that is okay and part of the human experience. It provided a pathway to work with discipline and devotion, to connect to my inner strength, fire, and faith. Studying yoga in India made me realize that God/Goddess does exist, that I am interconnected to all beings and to the universe, that there is peace available and embodied already within me, and that I am good enough just as I am.

Feeling *good enough just as I am* was a complete game changer, my friend.

We live in a world that is hell-bent, whether consciously or unconsciously, on convincing us that we need to look different, be different, act different, do less or more, be less or more—and only then will we be accepted and find happiness. Systems of oppression thrive by intentionally marginalizing certain groups and making them feel lesser than. There are all these -isms and phobias—capitalism, racism, sexism, classism, ableism, heterosexism, transphobia, xenophobia, and more—that are human-made and hold us back on a daily basis.

We must become aware, strong, resilient, and fill our hearts and minds with love and compassion to dismantle these systems of inequity and reimagine new ways of being in worlds where everyone is treated as an equal and there is no hierarchy of beings.

In my work as a trauma-informed yoga teacher and mindfulness educator, I have seen how many of us feel this sense of disconnection, self-loathing, anxiety, depression, and loneliness. It breaks my heart time after time to hear the teens I work with at mental health centers say things like "I hate my nose," "I prefer when people say mean things to me," or "I'm not good at anything." Meanwhile, the women of color who I have had the greatest honor of having as my private yoga clients have cried in sessions with me. Cried over feeling like they don't have a connection to their culture and traditions. Cried because they couldn't speak their mother tongue. Cried because they felt broken and didn't know how to heal. Cried because they felt caught between worlds and cultures.

There is a deep disconnect in the world today, and people are hurting. This brokenness is evident in the alarming 62 percent increase in suicide rates among American youth ages 10 to 24 from 2007 to 2021, the growing number of mass shootings in the United States, and the rising number of people who experience loneliness every day.

For me, yoga was a path out of this brokenness. It gave me direction, devotion, and faith, and it led me back to Sikhism. And that is why I have written this book. Yoga strengthened my already present desire for all beings to be free and well.

I hope to give language to folks who have felt unseen, judged, excluded, or ostracized in modern yoga spaces—to assure them that it is not their fault and to help them process that sense of being "othered." This exclusion has been crafted through histories of appropriation by colonialism, white supremacy, capitalism, casteism, patriarchy, and fitness culture.

In this book, I touch on the true heart of yoga—as something for *everyone* if they choose it for themselves, as a pathway of self-realization, enlightenment, self-love and self-acceptance, healing, and transformation. As a pathway for the liberation of all beings.

The yoga space is diverse, with much debate and difference of opinion. In writing this book, I have tried to hold space for as much of that diversity as possible. However, this book reflects who I am, my perspectives, and who I have written this book for. It is important to acknowledge our identities and where we come from—this impacts our worldview and conscious and unconscious biases. I am a yoga practitioner, lifelong student, and teacher, and did not write this book as a historian or scholar. I did not write this book as an expert, only as someone sharing insights from my lived experiences. I identify as a daughter of working-class immigrants, Punjabi Sikh, American-born, bilingual, able-bodied, brown, queer, straight-passing, middle-class, college-educated, thirty-one-year-old cis woman born and raised in California. I hold identities of both privilege and marginalization. I know I experience privilege due to being able-bodied, being cis and straight-passing, and because of my age, language fluency, college education, light skin, citizenship status, and socioeconomic class. I know I experience marginalization due to my gender, race, ethnicity, being a religious minority, and being the daughter of working-class immigrants, raised with economic hardship and limited social capital. These acknowledgments allow us to move through the world with more awareness—on how we can leverage our privilege for social change and acknowledging the injustices of the world that we have inherited.

My hope is that this book is a healing balm, so people have the words to express why the way yoga is taught isn't comprehensive and to know they are not alone in this feeling. To feel seen and heard. I wrote this book for myself, to the version of me from the past—and even the present—who feels left out.

I wrote this book for those of us who have walked into a modern yoga class and thought, How is this yoga? For those from the culture where yoga emerged, South Asia, who don't see ourselves represented in yoga spaces. Who don't see ourselves represented in the yoga magazines, in the yoga brands, at the studios, or at the festivals—to the ones who feel left out, erased, and not included.

For those of us who have a persistent feeling that the way that yoga is currently taught is surface level. For those of us who are seeking something "more real" but are not even sure what that means or looks like because we haven't had exposure to it.

I wrote this book for all the people of color, and particularly the women of color, who crave a connection to their motherland, to their healing practices, to their spiritual practices, and to a sense of community. A connection to something that might have gotten lost or stolen through colonialism, capitalism, assimilation, patriarchy, or forced conformity. This book is for the global majority who want to reclaim the connection to their roots, culture, and ancestral practices. Living in this modern world while seeking tradition, culture, and rituals to anchor us back to ourselves, one another, earth and nature, the universe, God/Goddess, our ancestors, and the divine.

To the white or privileged yoga practitioners who know there must be a better way, to those from the dominant culture, and maybe even to those who have unknowingly participated in appropriation in the past: This is a book for you too. This book is a loving call-in and is not about shaming or blaming. It is a call to understand and then to do better and be a participant in collective healing.

I want us all to have and feel a spiritual connection through the practice of yoga. To grow mentally, spiritually, and emotionally, and to grow our perspectives. To rebuild connections with ourselves, other beings, and this earth that is our home. I think yoga offers this pathway and transformation—but not the exercise method ruled by white supremacy, which wants to make it all about money, self-promotion, and exclusion. I think the true heart of yoga teaches love, a caring for the suffering of beings, and is a holding space for all emotions, nonviolence, and interconnectedness. I want the ones who want to embody that to learn and integrate it. To heal.

I recognize that yoga is not the answer to everything. The way yoga is practiced, taught, and portrayed is a symptom of what is happening at a larger scale. Modern-day yoga practice focused only on personal self-care will not solve systemic issues—this passes the responsibility from the collective to the individual. Ronald E. Purser shared in his book, *McMindfulness: How Mindfulness Became the New Capitalist Spirituality*, "Anything that offers success in our unjust society without trying to change it is not revolutionary—it just helps people cope." **Yoga practice can be a helpful tool, but it's not enough. A real revolution needs to address the root causes of suffering, not just teach people to cope with them.** Personal yoga practice is not going to solve all the systems of oppression; however, my hope is that it provides a pathway for personal liberation. There is a reason that certain lineages end by dedicating the merits of their efforts and practice to the liberation of all beings. We must attune ourselves toward being of service.

In this book, I use personal stories, historical insights, and analysis to understand how we have to come to this place with modern yoga. I intend this book to ask questions, not just provide solutions, and to be read as a reflective book. Take your time. My belief is that the answers will come from honest self-inquiry and contemplation.

Whoever you are, thank you for picking up this book. I wish for all beings to be happy, healthy, safe, and at ease. That includes you. Yoga is one path to get there. May we all find healing and true peace. And may this book be a (small) way to make that possible.

***

Reclaiming H(om)e

I reside on this land that I call home,
a land that my ancestors came to in the search and hope of better life,
their original home plundered and colonized.
Now I stand with one foot in this land,
of perceived freedom and opportunity
and one foot in the land of my ancestors—one of lush fields, spices, laughter, and community.
I'm from Panjab—The Land of Five Waters.
I'm the daughter to immigrants that only know survival.
I'm from ancient traditions and intricate rituals.
From a place where women are oppressed. Where my liberation is perceived as a threat.
I'm from a land of cha as love and marigolds as God.
A yearning to return to land where my mother tongue is spoken in every corner.
But when I return, I still feel
like I do not completely belong.
The way I walk and talk immediately gives me away.
Not from here.
Not from there.
Straddling two worlds.
A foot in this land and one foot in that land.
Then I realize through practice,
true home abides within me, not somewhere external to me.
This remembering that I am always whole, always complete.
And I have yoga to thank for that.

1

MY SEARCH FOR BELONGING

FOR MOST OF my life, I felt like I didn't belong anywhere. When I was growing up, my Indian cousins and other extended family saw me as American and not "Indian enough," while American friends and other students in my classes thought of me as Indian and not American. I'm sure many folks of the global majority have been asked the question "No, but where are you *really* from?" It felt like I was living within the *hyphen* of being Punjabi-American or Indian-American. Not Indian enough because I had an American accent and grew up in the US but not American enough because I was not white. It's this in-between feeling like you're not entirely one identity or another.

This is a common feeling among those of us from the diaspora. The term *diaspora* refers to the dispersion or scattering of a particular group of people from their original homeland or ancestral territory to other parts of the world. The diaspora can occur "voluntarily" as communities seek better opportunities or escape from persecution, or it can be forced through circumstances like war, climate change, or colonization.

As a first-generation Indian American, I have felt caught between worlds. And growing up in America, I felt like I had to hide my differences, to conform and assimilate as best I could. This showed up in not wanting to take the lunches my mom cooked me to school—lunches of roti and dal. I didn't want the other kids to look over, wrinkle their noses in disgust, and ask what in the world I was eating.

I remember as a five-year-old trying to convince my parents that Santa Claus comes down the chimney in the middle of the night and leaves presents under the tree. They walked me over to the fireplace and showed me how the top of the fireplace was closed off and there would be no way big, jolly old Santa Claus could possibly fit down the chimney. My parents weren't trying to be grinches, but they had only arrived in the US ten years prior and had never celebrated Christmas before. This was a foreign (Christian) holiday to them, and they simply didn't understand!

When kids at school were talking about Britney Spears and NSYNC, I was bopping along to Bollywood songs. I felt this pressure to constantly change myself and morph into someone more culturally acceptable around my American friends to seem like I belonged. I found myself pretending that, yes, I too had listened to the latest Backstreet Boys song.

The first time I went to Punjab, India, as a nine-year old, my younger cousin Amana, then seven, teased me mercilessly about how I spoke and pronounced Punjabi. She repeated everything I said with a jeer and told me how poorly I spoke Punjabi. It took several years to realize I didn't speak Punjabi poorly; I just spoke it with an American accent!

When my parents would take me to gurdwaras, temples, and pujas, I was full of questions about why a certain ritual was being done. Many different reasons! Why did we cover our heads to go into the gurdwara? To show respect in the presence of those we revere. The top of the head is also called the Dasam Duar, or the tenth gate, a sacred place on the human body, and it is good to keep it covered as protection. Why did we need to sit through the Shabad Kirtan (communal singing of hymns from Sri Guru Granth Ji)? To help the mind find a state of calm and eternal optimism (Chardi Kala), experience internal peace, and merge with God through devotional singing.

Our Name as Divine Representations

My longing to belong showed up in sitting on my bed, hands in prayer pose in front of my chest, eyes scrunched closed, at the age of nine, praying that when I grew up, I would have blue eyes and blond hair. Oh, how I hold that younger version of me with such love and care.

My desire to belong as a kid showed up in wishing on a daily basis that I had an "American" name like Ashley or Sophia, so when teachers paused while reading the roll call, I wouldn't know it was going to be immediately followed by a hesitant "Har-pen-ter?" And I would shrink down in my seat and just nod, not correcting them.

My fifth grade English teacher, whom I ended up adoring (and who encouraged me to keep writing!), asked on the first day of school, "Do I pronounce it Harp-in-der or Har-pin-der?"

I shyly responded, "Either way works."

She looked at me with such assuredness and said, "It's your name; you tell me how you prefer to hear it and want it to be pronounced."

In my ten years of existence, no one had given me such authority over myself or expressed such an interest in hearing from me how to pronounce my name correctly.

I thought about it and responded, "Harp-in-der is how I prefer it."

She smiled. "Well then, Harp-in-der it is."

At that moment, I felt pride in my name. Something I had not felt my entire life. I felt truly seen. Something so simple as someone wanting to hear the correct pronunciation of my name.

For those of us with "different" or more "complicated" names, we get used to hearing it wrong and not correcting people. I know I did for most of my life. It brought with it lots of shame and embarrassment. I wished my parents had chosen an easier name that everyone knew how to pronounce. Because of my name and apparent otherness, I was bullied at school. And with a last name like Mann, I heard things like "Ooh, are you a man?!"

Around me, I saw other Indian, Chinese, and Arab kids choosing to go with more Western-sounding names like Bobby, Mo, or Elizabeth to fit in better. This feeling of being othered and not belonging starts so young for so many of us. Especially for those that come from a background or culture not in the "dominant culture" of the United States.

It took twenty-four years of being alive to learn to accept my name and then another two years to love it. Harpinder in Punjabi means *God's home*, where divinity resides. Where this is belonging. There's irony to searching outside of myself for belonging when my name itself represents the home of the divine. So that's what I was looking for in yoga: another way to love myself as I was. A way to connect to my culture and who I truly was. Perhaps—though I didn't realize it at the time—I was looking for a way to reconnect to the ancestral spirituality and even religion of my source culture.

Sikhism's Ethical and Service-Oriented Foundation

Growing up, I was raised in a traditional Punjabi Sikhi household that also believed in Hinduism and revered Durga Mata. My grandparents would share stories about the Sikh Gurus and all the ways that they would fight for good and justice. From my bibiji and dadaji (grandmother and grandfather), I heard about Sikh gurus who believed in practicing gender equality, eliminating caste, being of selfless service (seva), working honestly (kirat karo), sharing with all beings for the highest good (vand chakko), and treating all people well, no matter their position in the world. That left an impact on me, and it informed my worldview.

I learned that in 1699 CE, Guru Gobind Singh declared that all men initiated into Sikhism would be given the name Singh, meaning *lion*, and all women who were initiated would be given the name Kaur, meaning *princess* or *lioness*. This indicated the removal of caste and represented equality within all of humanity. (I acknowledge the erasure of nonbinary and trans folks in this act.)

My bibiji shared a story about Guru Nanak Dev Ji, who traveled many places and was visiting a town called Saidpur. Word spread that a holy man was going to visit the town. In this town lived a corrupt governor named Malik Bhago, who earned a lot of wealth through unfair means. He would cheat poor farmers, leaving them hungry. Malik assumed Guru Ji would stay at his palace, and he began preparations for his arrival. However, when Guru Nanak reached Saidpur, he chose to stay with a poor carpenter named Lalo, who served Guru Ji with what little he had to offer, and Guru Ji ate the simple food with love. Malik heard about this and got angry—he ordered Guru Ji to his palace, and Guru Ji decided to go.

Malik Bhago said, "Oh holy man, I have prepared so many dishes for you, but you are staying with a lowly carpenter and eating his stale bread. Why?"

The guru responded, "I cannot eat your food because it has been made with money sucked from the poor through unfair means, while Lalo's food is made from hard-earned and honest money." Guru Ji proved his point by squeezing both men's bread: sweet honey dripped out from Lalo's bread, while blood dripped from Malik Bhago's bread. The nectar of honesty versus the blood of exploitation. Malik Bhago, shaken, asked for forgiveness. Upon Guru Ji's advice, he was instructed to share his ill-gotten wealth with the underprivileged and commit to a life of honesty. Malik Bhago was reborn under the guru's blessing and began leading an honest life.

These ethics and morals are the foundation for these teachings and provide guidance on how we can all live an honest life, making the world better for all beings. My grandparents told me stories about Sikhi warriors, gurus, and saints who had such courage and faith and had supernatural powers. Who stood up for what they believed in, even if for some gurus, it cost them and their families their lives. In their stories, I learned how Sikhs have faced violence and oppression since the beginning.

I was also surrounded by my parents and family members who would devoutly pray every morning without fail, go to temple every Sunday, and talk about God and how anything is possible with this support. Devotion, love, and surrender to God (bhakti) were prominently featured in my upbringing. This is what I came to associate bhakti yoga with—this reverence, devotion, and faith.

Every morning, I would shove my face deep under my blankets to hide from the smell of the incense my mom would offer to the pictures of Guru Nanak and Guru Ram Dass hanging on the walls of my room. I could hear her reciting parts of the Japji Sahib, known as the Mool Mantar, almost under her breath.

> ੧ੴ ਸਤਿ ਨਾਮੁ ਕਰਤਾ ਪੁਰਖੁ ਨਿਰਭਉ ਨਿਰਵੈਰੁ ਅਕਾਲ ਮੂਰਤਿ
> ਅਜੂਨੀ ਸੈਭੰ ਗੁਰ ਪ੍ਰਸਾਦਿ ॥
> *Ik-oa’nkār*
> There is only One God
> *sat̲ nām*
> Truth is his name
> *kart̲ā purakẖ nirbẖa-o nirvair akāl mūrat̲*
> He is the creator: without fear; without hate; he is immortal, without form
> *ajūnī saibẖa’n*
> Never born, self-perpetuating, he is self-illuminated
> *gur parsāḏ*
> He is realized by the kindness of the true Guru.
> —Śrī Guru Granth Sāhib Jī, *Japjī*, Mūl Mantār

This was a ritual I grew accustomed to expecting every single morning at six o'clock. I don't think there is a day my mom missed, even when feeling unwell. This devotion and faith run deep into the very core of one's being.

However, by the time I was preparing to leave for university, I had pushed Sikhism and religion away. My parents had a dogmatic approach of *believe it because we say so* that didn't feel right, and their actions didn't always match their stated values. While Sikhism speaks of gender equality, Punjabi culture still holds onto patriarchal values.

My parents placed gender roles onto me, saying that girls cooked and cleaned so that they would be prepared to do so for their future husband and in-laws. I remember as a nine-year-old exclaiming, "Will his hands be broken? Why will I be responsible for all of it?"

Sikhism teaches about seva to care for and protect all beings through conquering self-centered desires and behaviors. However, my family faced physical and verbal abuse at the hands of my dad, who felt we were not on his side. This wreaked terror into our lives daily. No child should ever have to witness and experience such abuse and violence. Because of my dad's increasing paranoia that people were after him, including my mom, we moved to five different cities in five years, each time leaving me, my mom, and two brothers to have to deal with the ramifications. I attended four different middle schools, and as an awkward, shy 10-year-old, making new friends felt like a herculean task each time I arrived halfway through the school year. Talk about feeling like you don't belong!

Several times a week, I would pray to God that my dad would stop hurting us and he would see the world clearly. But God didn't seem to listen, and slowly I lost my faith. I felt the cognitive dissonance of my dad acclaiming himself as such a godly man and then doing such horrific things, and I thought, How could God really exist if such horror is permitted in the world? What kind of God is this? At that time, I couldn't separate the two. I felt my only recourse was to ostracize myself from all of it completely. To become a nonbeliever.

An Outsider's Perspective at UCLA

By the time I landed at the University of California, Los Angeles, I was grateful to have space to become my own person and shape my life as I saw fit. Having accessed freedom for the first time, away from the (overly) watchful eyes of my parents, I turned heavily to partying. This became my outlet to celebrate, grieve, connect, socialize, and feel liberated. However, binge drinking and drugs, while cathartic in the moment, did nothing to help me make sense of my life and my direction. Thus, at UCLA, I still felt lost and out of place. It makes me think of the quote from *Buckaroo Banzai*, "No matter where you go, there you are." I had to find a way to work with my mind.

The high school I had attended did not prepare me for the rigors of university—one of my classmates shared casually how her high school courses were more difficult than her UCLA classes. As someone who had barely passed her first quarter at UCLA after putting in countless all-nighters, drinking copious amounts of coffee, and turning to "smarter" students for study help, I was shocked. At my high school in the Central Valley, I was one of only two people who got into UCLA from a class of over four hundred people. I had graduated as valedictorian, at the top of my class and with the most community service hours completed (seva embodied). My school was mostly made up of Latine people, followed by white people, and then with smaller percentages of Asian and Black people. At UCLA, I was struck by the number of white people and by the number of students who clearly had money. Students drove BMWs, Mercedes, and Range Rovers and spoke about international vacations.

As someone who was born lower-middle class, this was a huge adjustment. I was paying my own way through UCLA and juggling school, a work-study job that paid eight dollars an hour, an unpaid internship, and student activism.

In comparison, I felt less-than, behind, and like an ugly duckling. I was taught by my family to work hard, twice as hard as my American counterparts, and that I had to take care of myself because no one else would. That left a mark on me. I felt like I always had to keep pushing, succeeding, because no one was coming to save me or even help me.

My experience is not unique. Many people share similar stories. Second-generation immigrants like me may be at higher risk of poor mental health due to the demands associated with navigating two cultures and feelings of not belonging in the immigrant culture or the host population.

I knew I needed something to help anchor me. The partying was not going to be the solution. There was a stirring within me, a need to reconnect to spirit, God/Goddess, universe, anything larger than myself that could support me. And I had the faint sense that yoga also had something to do with spirituality, with being that bridge or connection, easing anxiety, bringing harmony and peace.

I went on a search for yoga because there was a part of me that knew I wasn't less-than. But covertly, those were the messages I was receiving and feeling. I was looking for something to make me feel whole. To feel less anxious. To feel settled in my skin.

Unfortunately, that's not what I found in the first yoga classes I attended.

My First Yoga Classes in Los Angeles: Yoga Shared as Exercise

"NAAAMASTE!"

I jolted slightly in my cross-legged position on my borrowed yoga mat. As I peeked around my hands, held in front of me in prayer pose, I observed people bowing down to the instructor, who was sitting at the front. The thin, white, cis female instructor clad in leggings and a sports bra quickly got up and left the room without a glance back at us. The loud exclamation of "namaste" at the end of class was perhaps the only marker that this was not just a modern fitness class taking place in a sweaty, heated, fogged-up room but also a practice that had *some* connection to India and, more broadly, to South Asia.

But what *was* that connection? And why did I still feel a bit uneasy, like I did not belong in this space, even though my family had immigrated to the United States from Punjab, India, less than thirty years ago?

I had made my way to this class at CorePower Yoga studio in Westwood, California, in 2013 as a sophomore at UCLA. One of the first things I noticed walking into the studio was how out of place I both felt and looked. All around me were conventionally attractive, fit, and youthful people dressed in color-coordinated, tight-fitting clothing, with labels like Lululemon, Alo Yoga, and Nike predominantly featured. I wore baggy black shorts and the oversized, wrinkled "Go Bruins" shirt I had received for free at orientation. I immediately felt myself shrinking in comparison to everyone else, trying and failing to smooth down the frizz in my hair that I had pulled into a ponytail.

I tentatively looked around at the beginning of class, hoping to find someone who looked like me, and was met with only white faces.

Over the course of the next sixty minutes—in a room so steamy I could barely see the person on the mat in front of me, with all twenty of us squeezed in like sardines, and with pop music pumping from speakers—the instructor led us from pose to pose with efficiency and speed. I barely had time to catch my breath or connect with my physical body. By the time we arrived in savasana, I felt great relief in being able to lie down and collect myself. I did feel some sense of peace—that I was able-bodied enough to mostly follow along and could now finally rest.

However, I had come to this class hoping to make connections with the teacher and other students and to learn how yoga might help with the existential dread and anxiety I was experiencing. I was looking for life guidance and support. Instead, I got a heart-pumping workout where I couldn't make sense of which way my limbs were flailing as I tried to keep up.

I remember going back to my roommates and saying, "If yoga is just all about exercise, I prefer running and lifting weights!"

What a shame that I walked away with this impression when there is so much more to yoga, so much more depth and potential for transformation and a return to wholeness.

In another yoga studio that I visited, YogaWorks, I was relieved that at least there were only a few people in the class and that there was ample space to move and breathe. I was still the only person of color in the class of five. The class was titled "Gentle Flow," yet it still felt like there was an urgency in moving from pose to pose. At one point, the thin, white instructor came behind me, put her hands on my hips, and pulled me more into a V-shape in Downward-Facing Dog (Adho Mukha Svanasana). I felt shocked that someone adjusted me with such force without even asking if it was okay to touch me!

As a survivor of domestic violence and sexual abuse, I felt violated. The nonconsensual touch from the instructor made me feel queasy and icky. It also felt like a note to me that I was doing it wrong and needed to be better or different. That's what happens when the only note or feedback you receive the entire sixty-minute class is where you could be "better."

There was never any mention of the roots of yoga or its true goals, where this practice originated from, or what we were working toward other than toned, flexible bodies.

For anyone looking into these studios, I'm not sure how you would be able to tell the difference between this being a yoga class and a fitness class. Each studio I went to had a sterile feel, with white walls and wood floors. All the teachers were thin, white, cis, female, and able-bodied. In my search, I was able to find only studios like these, which taught yoga as exercise.

I felt even more lost and confused when I attended the yoga classes in the studios around Westwood, where UCLA is located. There was no mention of any philosophy, no explanation given. Nobody I met at the yoga studios seemed to care about me.

I went in seeking wise counsel and walked away with sore legs and a desire to purchase cuter workout clothes so that I could fit in (with money that I did not have!).

Where in these spaces was the thread of connection to spirituality and deeper meaning that I was seeking so desperately? Over the span of a year and a half, I went to more than a dozen studios and never found anything that felt right or *real*. Instead, I would find more of the same, that is, being the only person of color or one of just a few people of color in class—including staff and instructors. Yoga practiced as a workout and diluted down to asana as a sport with the aim of perfecting poses and showcasing flexibility as competition. Sanskrit terms used without explanation, context, or understanding. Statues and pictures of Hindu gods and goddesses used merely as decoration, placed in studio bathrooms and on the floor.

I was searching for yoga philosophy and for yoga as a way of being. I wanted a teacher, a mentor, *someone* to help guide me as a directionless nineteen-year-old. I associated yoga, and more specifically bhakti yoga, with what I was raised with in my family with Sikhism, with the devotion, prayer, and guidance on how to live life ethically. However, in this modern yoga scene, I found something very different. Still, I kept going to different studios in this search because, even though I knew there was more beyond the asana than was being practiced, I felt myself becoming stronger physically and did experience a bliss state in savasana—something I don't think I had ever experienced in my life before. There was a sparkle, a glimmer of peace there. A turning in I wasn't finding in other spaces, in other areas of my life. I kept searching because even in these fitness-oriented asana classes, I still felt something. A stirring and awakening within of something deeper, a sense of *there is something here*, and I needed to keep investigating. However, I still didn't entirely feel like I belonged in these yoga studios.

As humans, we are hardwired to want to belong. This is an innate and universal aspect of human nature. And to search for a place that feels safe and like home, a place where you belong, are accepted, and are loved, can be a difficult process. This search brought me to many different places. The original ache of *not belonging* that I was hoping to resolve had taken me to yoga in the first place. Eventually, I gave up going to yoga studios because what I was truly seeking was not there. I was hoping to gain a spiritual practice.

State of Modern Yoga in the West

This is largely the state of modern yoga now in the West:

It has been whitewashed and sterilized to the point that yoga is grossly equated to a workout. There is frequently no acknowledgment that there is more to yoga than just stretching and contorting the body. Many yoga influencers, teachers, and practitioners don't know or care to learn that yoga is a spiritual practice and path that originates from the Indian subcontinent with a very specific goal of liberation or moksha.

Yoga has been over-exoticized, culturally appropriated, and commodified. T-shirts are sold with sacred deities like Ganesha on them, sold and worn by people with no understanding of who Ganesha is. We have events like "Beer Yoga" and "Goat Yoga," and teachers enthusiastically tell their students to "nama-slay" the poses.

In the early years of my practice, I did not have the words to name what I was seeing, only the vague, persistent feeling that something about this was not right. Since then, I have come to know that what I was seeing and experiencing was the result of decades of colonization, cultural appropriation, and commodification.

How did we get here? And why is it important to recall and acknowledge yoga's roots and history?

How we got here is something I'll discuss throughout this book. As for the why: it's important to return to yoga's roots because the appropriated form of yoga was not something that could solve my problem of feeling disconnected from myself—if anything, it caused more disconnection and disorientation.

And that form of yoga can't help anyone else with their problems either.

Ultimately, yoga became a path of homecoming, to my roots and to my ancestral practices. It became a sanctuary in the truest sense of the word. I found my way to spaces where teachers who looked like me talked about the true goals of yoga and what that means for us as human beings reincarnated at this time, what our true purpose is. These teachers created real community and connection, got to know their students, and led me into yoga practice with more understanding around asana's importance. In these spaces, I found healing. I found a sense of belonging. I found knowledge that turned into wisdom on how to live my life.

However, I didn't find this path through yoga as it is commonly practiced in the West. For that, I had to return to my motherland of India.

2

RECONNECTING TO YOGA'S ROOTS

IT WASN'T UNTIL I started going to the Ananda Sangha center in New Delhi, India, in 2016 that I truly found a yoga community that felt holistic and *real*.

I was working as a director of business development and marketing for an education consulting start-up, and at times I felt in over my head. My role consisted of promoting the company to students and parents who needed assistance with college applications and bringing them on as new clients. A lot of our clients were in India, so this meant we would often travel to different parts of India—Bangalore, Delhi, Lucknow, Hyderabad, Jaipur, and more—to host in-person events. There were whole months when I lived in a hotel in India, giving my all for this company.

But I was plagued by impostor syndrome. I doubted my skills, talents, and accomplishments, and I constantly worried that I would be exposed as a fraud. This was combined with working for a CEO who demanded perfection and lacking colleagues to express my thoughts and concerns to. My impostor syndrome and anxiety only seemed to get worse while working in India, away from my support system. It slowly started to take a toll on my mental health.

There would be days when I felt like an elephant was sitting on my chest, and I was unable to take a full breath. Other days, I had a sensation of a lump of coal in my stomach, burning my insides, causing my hands to sweat with nervousness and anticipation of something bad happening. I felt this pull of needing to find something to help me. To feel settled in my skin, to feel a sense of peace within myself. To alleviate the anxiety.

I'm sure many people who have turned to yoga can relate to seeking this path and practice to help them feel better. I love the way Indu Arora states this: "The taste of sattva (purity) never starts with sweetness, but usually starts with bitter (realizations)."

An "aha" moment came to me when I realized, *I am in India now!* One of the birthplaces of yoga. Surely, I would find something real here. Google searches brought me to the Ananda Sangha center in New Delhi. The center's website stated, "Ananda is dedicated to the belief, born of experience, that you can live in joy. We teach effective techniques for expanding your sense of self, such as meditation, spiritual Hatha yoga, and divine friendship."

Now *this*—this sounded more real to me.

My First Yoga Class in New Delhi: Yoga Shared as a Spiritual Practice

One evening, I called a cab and headed over to the center. It took twenty minutes to reach the center, and as I got out of the cab and walked through the gates, I was taken aback by the lush plants surrounding the building. Around the walkway were sculptures of an om and a cross, white statues of people seated in lotus posture with flower garlands around their necks, and deep orange marigold flowers decorating the doorway.

I took my shoes off outside, and as I crossed the threshold, I was greeted warmly by a gentleman in his early thirties. He asked my name and showed me to the room where we would be practicing asana. I felt every muscle in my body relax as I looked at the space around me. There were shelves full of books, a warmth emanated from the building itself, and it felt like I had finally arrived.

I immediately felt accepted and welcomed.

When I sat down on the carpet of the room we were practicing in, the teacher smiled gently at me and asked, "How are you doing today, beti?" At that moment, I felt seen and cared for. She was an older woman in her sixties, with shoulder-length gray hair, and wore glasses and a traditional Punjabi and Pakistani outfit of a salwar kameez (long tunic with comfortable pants). Imagine, a yoga teacher not in a matching spandex set.

The first five to ten minutes were spent with everyone getting settled into their seats and talking to one another, welcoming any new people with big smiles and warm introductions. I noticed that I was the youngest person by at least fifteen to twenty years. The woman sitting next to me smiled and remarked in Hindi, "It's so good you're learning yoga so young! Please keep coming back."

When we began practicing, the asana practice was gentle, with a focus on healing affirmations. There was no race from one pose to another, nor the instruction to contort the body quickly like it was an acrobatics competition. An intentionality of moving slowly and steadily was offered and created throughout the practice. We would spend two to three minutes in parivrtta sukhasana (easy seated twist) on each side. We were cued to notice where our eyes were focusing, to notice the quality of our breath, and then affirmation was offered: "I radiate love and goodwill to soul friends everywhere." A feeling of ease settled over me.

Each time I came back to the center, different people would ask how I was doing. There was never a sense of *we know better than you at the center* but an ample space created for self-inquiry and introspection to happen. For my curiosity to be accepted and applauded. There was space to ask questions and space to turn into myself with gentleness and compassion. I don't think I'd ever experienced or been taught this before. To hold myself gently, even in the midst of confusion and doubt. Over the next few months of coming to this center, I was struck by how it and its teachers exuded warmth and humility. There were never more than six people in the class, and the room was cozy, with carpet throughout and with pictures of self-realized gurus like Paramahansa Yogananda, whose book *Autobiography of a Yogi* I was encouraged to read. The book struck me. I was taken by Yogananda's description of his encounter with his guru, Swami Sri Yukteswar, who was levitating several inches off the floor while in meditation! This made me feel that there is so much more potential to me that I didn't even know about. There were also images of Swami Kriyananda, Jesus Christ, Sri Yukteswar, Lahiri Mahasaya, and Mahavatar Babaji on the walls. I appreciated and welcomed the recognition of the enlightened beings regardless of religion.

The teachers taught with care, devotion, and a deep focus on realizing God/Goddess and our profound connection to spirit and all beings. Here I experienced Kriya Yoga, kirtan, meditation, and satsangs where teachers shared yogic philosophy. There were discussions on topics like karma, seva, ethics, contentment, death, self-realization, the shedding of all outward self-definitions, and the integration of spirituality into one's life.

This was what I had been searching for. Yes, I was looking for the practices, but I was also looking for the wisdom and teachings to make sense of my life. I was looking for a community where we could have discussions on how to work with the mind, with emotions, and integrate these teachings into my life. I wanted to understand the ethical and moral underpinnings of yoga, the psychological framework to work with my mind, and the teachings to use as wisdom in my life.

Over the course of several months, I found what had been missing in the modern yoga classes: yoga shared as a spiritual practice—a path and practice as a way of life to help reduce suffering and ultimately work toward self-realization and liberation; the experiential understanding that we are connected to something greater than ourselves and to ultimately merge with the divine; how this practice of yoga allows us to experience the radical truth that we are all worthy and equal. I finally felt and understood yoga as a gateway to access our internal self, purusha, which is whole, infinite, and perfect.

In the taxi ride back to my hotel after these classes, with tears of gratitude running down my cheeks, I felt something deep within me change forever. It was this embodied sense that I am part of something larger, that I was in harmony with the natural world around me. A doorway to my self had been opened that led me to an experience of a unity that transcends all boundaries and encompasses all beings. Mystics, poets, artists, and yogis in every age have spoken of this unity as the highest truth, and I finally was able to access it.

I remember looking out of the window during the taxi rides I took after every class I went to and sensing that a profound knowing was being unlocked—one of peace, contentment, and joy. A knowing that all this exists within me and that, through practice, I could access this peace, contentment, and joy. *There is nothing I need to purchase or externally achieve to access this state.* It comes through devotion, discipline, and deep listening. By simply being, I am divine. To acutely touch and feel this inner peace forever altered the course of my life.

When I first sought out the yoga class in Westwood, although I didn't exactly know it at the time, I was seeking a connection to my homeland of Punjab, to my culture, to spirituality, and to my healing ancestral practices. I was seeking answers to questions like, *What is my purpose? What is the meaning of life? How do I find fulfillment and happiness? Is there a way to alleviate this existential angst and anxiety? Is there more to life than this? How do I make a positive difference in this world?*

Yoga helps us to answer these questions. It provides a pathway. However, this context and depth is missing in modern asana classes like those I encountered in California. Practicing yoga at the Ananda Sangha center was like a balm for my soul. Finally, I had found a place where I could both intellectually and experimentally begin to understand these things and where I would be held with the loving support of community.

When I returned to Los Angeles, I found an Ananda Sangha center in Larchmont (this no longer exists) and started attending classes, sometimes four or five times a week. There was a mix of offerings of practice, education, and discussion. In one of the classes, the teacher described in great length the five koshas (originating from the Taittiriya Upanishad), the five sheaths or layers encasing the pure consciousness (purusha) or Self (atman). They are known as the annamaya kosha (food sheath), pranamaya kosha (prana, or life force, sheath), manomaya kosha (mind sheath), vijnanamaya kosha (wisdom sheath), and anandamaya kosha (bliss sheath).

Learning this made me realize how much more there is to us as human beings beyond just the physical body and mind, and how different practices help us to transcend each layer and tune into the true nature of the Self. For instance, with the vijnanamaya kosha, it is learning that you are more than your intellect and ability to analyze. The study of scriptures, right inquiry (Who am I?), and meditation are all common methods to quiet the churning of the mind and travel beyond the limitations of intellect. These koshas are like peeling away the layers of an onion to get to the truth and heart of our beingness, which is the divine Self.

It's a reminder that we are not these limited beings we take ourselves to be. As an eager and sincere student, I was hungry for knowledge and wisdom that helped me to know myself better. To understand the world better.

During my first experience of restorative yoga, the teacher told me that the most important part of practice was being as comfortable as possible. She layered blankets underneath my knees, supported my ankles, enveloped me with more blankets, and slowly placed an eye pillow on my face. I still recall to this day how my nervous system completely settled and how cared for I felt. I have so much love and admiration for yoga teachers who tend to their students in this way.

In Buddhism, there is the concept of taking refuge in the Triple Gem, or the Three Jewels. This is taking refuge in Buddha as the example, the dharma (the teachings), and the sangha (the community of practitioners). Taking refuge is a way to formalize one's commitment and faith in the Buddha's path and potential for liberation. This also translates to yoga. Yoga and Buddhism are inexorably linked as they emerged in history at a parallel time, with shared roots, teachings, and practices. In the yoga tradition, the journey of seeking inner awakening has been lovingly guided and supported by the guru–shishya–shastra parampara. This is the threefold system of teacher–student–scriptures. The fourth I add to this is sangha, the community. It is important to have a guide or teacher as an example and as a transmitter, to have teachings to turn to for knowledge, and to be in a safe, loving community that supports you and encourages you, especially when you are struggling.

I wish for all seekers and students on this journey to be held by the path in this way. To have a teacher, the wisdom of the teachings, and a community, and where teachers on this path take this role and responsibility seriously and continue studying and growing.

Yoga Taught with Ethics, Philosophy, and Wisdom

In popular or modern yoga, it is too often the case that a selective portion of the teachings, the physical practices—the asana or poses—are extracted and then made to be the whole of what yoga is. What we really need is for these physical practices to be shared in harmony with the larger yogic teachings of ethics, philosophy, and wisdom. Otherwise, we do a disservice to the entire methodology. Even Buddhism gets reduced to mindfulness meditation when it is a whole tradition with many different schools and lineages such as Theravada, Mahayana, and Vajrayana.

As Dr. Miles Neale, Buddhist psychotherapist, shares in his piece, "On McMindfulness and Frozen Yoga: Rediscovering the Essential Teachings of Ethics and Wisdom," if we continue emphasizing the physical practice without the understanding of philosophical and psychological wisdom and ethics, we will get only temporary states of peace. These temporary states of peace, which we might experience at the conclusion of an asana class during savasana or while chanting "om," might feel nice in that moment but are not enough to reach the everlasting moksha (liberation) or dukha-nivritti (elimination of suffering) that traditional yoga refers to.

True freedom and liberation mean observing and eliminating any misperceptions that trigger reactive habits and cause harmful actions. This means to self-inquire and self-reflect on what types of habits you hold, how you conduct yourself with yourself and others, and if your beliefs and actions are causing harm. Yoga is not meant to be a self-serving path of spirituality where we don't think about our interconnectedness to everything and all beings. Yoga is an inner science (adhyatmavidya) that dives deep to transform your entire being, aiming to reshape your daily life, your perspective, and your very approach to the world.

In Dr. Shyam Ranganathan's commentary and translation of the Yoga Sutras of Patanjali, he speaks to these reactive habits and patterning (samskaras) that we hold in Sutra 2.12:

> *kleśa-mūlaḥ karmāśayo dṛṣṭādṛṣṭa-janma-vedanīyaḥ*
>
> *The root of affliction is past action. It is latent, seen or unseen, and stays with us through births in the form of experiences that produce further karma. If we wish to be rid of our present afflictions, we must find a way to sever the root that nourishes such affliction and yoga is the means.*

If we practice yoga asana to experience only temporary states of peace, we never get to the roots of our patterning or seek to change them. We have to allow yoga asana (as one means) to look deeply at ourselves and see where we have habits, patterning, and reactions (whether conscious or unconscious) that not only cause harm to ourselves but also to those around us. This is where we have to bring our negative samskaras into the light and investigate them—not as a way to punish or judge ourselves but as a way to acknowledge we are all imperfect beings with need of skillful refinement. As a way to admit that some patterning has come from previous lifetimes, from modeling from your parents, and from societal conditioning. Instead of pursuing yoga as solely a feel-good modality, we have to turn to its ethical and wisdom underpinnings as a vehicle for our own growth and transformation, which then transcends out all around us. This means to take yoga off the mat into every aspect of our life. This looks like deep study and contemplation on topics like selflessness, karma, seva, and consciousness.

I worry, similarly to others in this space, such as my teacher Dr. Miles Neale, that we are losing the deeper spiritual and philosophical aspects that underlie the practice of yoga and are watering down the essential ingredients of this liberation tradition. It is imperative that we reunite these practices with their original intents and goals so that yoga doesn't become something completely unrecognizable. And I think that is a role and responsibility for all people who call themselves students and teachers of yoga!

This requires deep study and integration of the philosophy of yoga, over many years, with no rush, and with a good teacher who can serve as a guide and mirror. It requires a commitment to studentship throughout life, to self-inquiry and refinement, and to being a student practitioner before you are a teacher. It requires self-awareness and the willingness to look at oneself honestly to make changes to become a more conscious, compassionate, and ethical being.

To understand the ethics of yoga, we can turn to Patanjali's yamas and niyamas (as one example) here:

ahiṃsā-satyāsteya-brahmacaryāparigrahā yamāḥ (2.30)

Yoga Sutra 2.30 says that the rules of moral conduct (yamas) are nonviolence (ahimsa), truthfulness (satya), not stealing (asteya), celibacy or "right use of energy" (brahmacharya), and nonattachment or non-greed (aparigraha). Ethical guidelines assist in cultivating mental integrity, curbing primal instincts, and providing a framework for the mind's operations. An ethically attuned mind is a regulated mind.

Becoming mindful of your beliefs and actions, having brave contemplative spaces to self-inquire, and knowing how interconnected we all are: **I think this will move us in the direction of true happiness and freedom.**

Ahimsa and the Middle Way

Since 2018, I have taught yoga one-on-one to folks of color who want to heal in a safe space and deepen their relationship to yoga in a way that honors the practice. I have sat on panels, virtually and in-person, at conferences and festivals where we spoke about what it looks like to decolonize yoga. I have taught and mentored aspiring yoga teachers and run workshops on dismantling cultural appropriation. In all these spaces, I get asked questions like the following:

- What are the true goals of yoga?
- There are so many different lineages and paths of yoga (that have different limbs and ideologies). Do I have to learn all of them?
- What is the history of yoga and where can I learn?
- What effect did the two-hundred-year-long colonization of India by the British Raj have on yoga?
- What is the difference between culturally appropriating and appreciating yoga?
- How do I practice with reverence?
- Is it unethical to charge for yoga classes?
- But what if I am interested in asana as only a workout, then what?

Here's the thing. For some of these questions, there is no resounding clear-cut answer. Rather, the way forward is through cultivating a greater understanding of the context and history of yoga. As a yoga and Buddhist/dharma practitioner, I have been taught ahimsa and the middle way, where ahimsa is the commitment to not to cause harm and the middle way is about not going toward either extreme. There is a need for pause and self-inquiry that might cause discomfort, discernment, and questioning.

The best thing we can ever say is, "I don't know, but I am willing to try to learn and find out." The best thing we can aim for is to be better than we were yesterday. I am reminded of Maya Angelou's quote: "Do the best you can until you know better. Then when you know better, do better."

This is all I encourage and ask in this book, from my students and from all sincere practitioners. I am not here to say people should stop practicing or teaching—far from it! Simply that all should broaden their understanding, to know that there is more.

I am humbled to be a steward in this way, to be a part of this very important conversation. Humbled and walking with gentleness because yoga is so expansive—with different traditions, practices, and lineages—and while there is no way I will ever be able to write about or even know all of it, this book comes from a special place within me. I am honored to write, create, and share something so necessary so that people can practice responsibly for the good of the world, their communities, and themselves. My ultimate hope is that as many people as possible will find their way to the path of rediscovering yoga's roots, which led me toward healing and freedom.

Before we dive into the rest of the book, I want to offer definitions of yoga that I personally attune to. It is important to remember that yoga is not a monolithic system. Because yoga originated in the Indic region, gaining a comprehensive understanding of yoga necessitates a careful examination of the fundamental beliefs, historical context, and cultural foundations, as well as the nuances of language and symbolism unique to that region, over the thousands of years that it evolved. It's also worth noting that yoga first originated as an oral tradition, so dating is not exact.

Seeing Clearly

Patanjali's Yoga Sutras defines yoga as "*yogaś citta-vṛtti-nirodhaḥ*" (1.2). This can be understood as "yoga is the restraint of the activities of the mind-stuff," "yoga is the stilling of the changing states of the mind," or "yoga is the quelling of the chaotic mind patterns."

We practice to arrive at a state where we have peace of mind, where we are able to perceive ourselves and the world clearly without disturbance or misperception. We want to eliminate the potential of rajas and tamas to allow the potential of the sattvic nature of the mind to manifest. This means to still the mind through meditative concentration on a particular object of choice without any distractions. In other words, we want to be able to focus our attention and mind as we please, without getting distracted.

According to Sankhya philosophy, all material objects are made of three gunas or *characteristics*. The three gunas are tamas, rajas, and sattva. Tamas is *inertia*, rajas is *dynamism* and sattva is *steadiness*. For example, a rock represents tamas, man represents rajas, and divinity represents sattva. The dull mind or the mind in which there is no awareness is tamasic or inert; the mind which oscillates between awareness and no awareness is rajasic or dynamic; and the steady, one-pointed mind is sattvic. It is said one who transcends tamas and rajas and is ruled by sattva is a great yogi.

By stilling our mind this way, we are able to reflect the true image of the soul to itself. Yoga Sutra 1.2 reminds us of the true purpose of yoga: for us to remember the nature of who we are—purusha, the eternal Self that is perfect, timeless, and complete. Sutra 1.3, *tadā draṣṭuḥ svarūpe 'vasthānam*, points to this realization—then in a state of yoga, the seer rests in its true nature. This realization tells us that we are enough, just as we are, and can rest in our beingness.

We attain this goal through several ways, as mentioned in the Yoga Sutras. In the first pada (chapter), Sutra 1.12, *abhyāsa-vairāgyābhyāṃ tan-nirodhaḥ*, Patanjali identifies two ingredients necessary for restraint of the vrittis: abhyasa (continuous practice) and vairagya (unattachment). They are like two wings of a bird; both are needed and incredibly important practices in yoga. Yatna (effort) is required for continuous practice. In Sutra 1.14, Patanjali teaches us that our practice needs to be cultivated uninterruptedly, over a long period of time, and with complete faith. This diligent practice, or sadhana, creates a firm foundation and helps us in transforming our mind, habits, and layers of ignorance. This is why self-work in yoga is understood to be an extensive process of dedication, sincerity, and vigor. We must remain dedicated and patient on this path, with both abhyasa and vairagya. It might be a lifetime(s) of dedicated work!

The other way the goal of Yoga is attained is through Kriya yoga, *tapaḥ-svādhyāyeśvara-praṇidhānāni kriyā-yogaḥ* (2.1), which refers to tapas (self-discipline and purification); svadhyaya (continuous, deep study of sacred wisdom and the introspective search into the nature of the self); and ishvara pranidhana (wholehearted devotion and dedication to Ishvara). This is laid out as a way to eliminate the kleshas, the obstacles to yoga, and to attain samadhi.

There is also the eight-limbed path, otherwise known as Ashtanga yoga, *yama-niyamāsana-prāṇāyāma-pratyāhāra-dhāraṇā-dhyānasamādhayo 'ṣṭāv aṅgāni* (2.29). The eight limbs are (1) yamas, or moral conduct; (2) niyamas, or observances; (3) asana, or posture; (4) pranayama, or practices to expand the dimensions of prana within you; (5) pratyahara, or withdrawal of the senses from their objects; (6) dharana, or on-pointed concentration; (7) dhyana, or meditation; and (8) samadhi, or absolute absorption. These offer further prescriptions for attaining the goal of yoga. It is important to practice them all. Yoga Sutra 2.28 says that by practicing the limbs of yoga, impurities are eliminated, wisdom arises, and clear-sighted awareness is cultivated.

Traditionally, the Yoga Sutras were not taught to beginners, unlike modern yogic trainings. Students used to study grammar, logic, syllogism, and Sankhya Darshana before coming to study the Yoga Sutras. On the other hand, the Bhagavad Gita is something a beginner student can be taught (by a teacher who has deeply studied it), as it speaks to a more lay audience (and to householders).

The Yoga Sutras go into the psychology and metaphysics of the yoga process and could possibly be the first manual of psychoanalysis and psychotherapy. It is a text on the science of the mind. This is why I think it is important to study this text with a good teacher. The original commentators of this text imagined students would have a background in Sankhya Darshana, the oldest systematically laid out philosophical model in Indian thought (ca. 800–700 BCE or even older). Sankhya covers purusha (pure awareness or consciousness) and prakriti (nature or matter, including the human mind and emotions). This school of thought covers suffering and how to come out of this bondage of suffering into liberation or moksha.

It is important to study Sankhya Darshana (philosophy) because it gives a framework for the study of yoga. We see it in texts like the Upanishads, the Mahabharata, and Patanjali's Yoga Sutras (and it provides a framework for Ayurveda as well). Also, many concepts that are fundamental to yoga, like the concept of gunas (sattva, rajas, and tamas), matter, and consciousness, et cetera, were first propagated by Sankhya metaphysics.

atha yogānuśāsanam (1.1)—Now, the teachings of yoga (are stated).

Here, the term *now* is significant because it is used in the sense of having accomplished something prior. It connotes that the study of the Yoga Sutras is picking up from where we left before (i.e., the study of Sankhya).

In the Yoga Sutra, Patanjali has addressed prakriti as "the seen" and purusha as "the seer." This is an easier way to understand that purusha is the fundamental knower, the subject, and prakriti is the fundamental known, the eternal creation, the object. To explain in simplistic terms, purusha is the real You—the true self—and Prakriti is all that is not really You, including your mind–body, car, house, job, et cetera.

The ultimate goal of yoga is described by various words such as kaivalya, samādhi, moksha, which is described as the experience of an individual soul uniting with the divine and/or becoming liberated from the material world.

As my teacher Sri Prasad Rangnekar shared during a Yoga Sutras course, "Sankhya tells us to experience the world (Prakriti), take what is relevant for self-growth, and continue the journey towards True Self (Purusha). It gives importance to one's experience and this is why it is empowering. We are all walking back home to our original pristine state of eternal Self. We are reminded here again that the process is going to take time, so be disciplined, motivated, patient and empathetic towards yourself. Yoga of Patanjali is all about Samadhi and all limbs of Ashtanga Yoga are steps to reach there."

So, let's begin.

3

ASANA AS FREEDOM FROM PHYSICAL FIXATION

A PROSPECTIVE PRIVATE client reached out to me by email, telling me about her issues and desires, asking whether I might be able to support her. She said that she had undergone physical therapy for lumbar and cervical spine sprains. Both her doctor and physical therapist had recommended stretching and yoga to her. She also hoped to focus on herself in 2022 because the last couple of years had been rough, with multiple deaths in her family.

Reading her email, I could empathize with her struggle. Several of the clients I had worked with had come to me after enduring physical injuries or ailments and being advised to take up yoga, while others similarly were looking to finally put themselves first.

In my reply, I sent her my well wishes and set up the first consultation call. During our conversation, she shared with me: "I am looking for someone to help me heal my back and feel better. I hurt my back while working, and my physical therapist recommended I try yoga. I went to a few yoga classes in the area, and I couldn't keep up. The instructor kept moving the class along quickly, and she never came over to tell me if I was doing it right or not. Aren't teachers supposed to help? I didn't feel noticed or acknowledged at all in those classes! Will you be able to help me?"

Again, this was something I had heard many times before from potential private clients. People would tell me that while they had certain physical injuries, differences, or disabilities, they didn't feel accounted for and weren't given accommodations to help them follow along. Most mainstream asana classes at yoga studios and gyms are catered to able-bodied folks. This excludes many people who are interested in getting into yoga asana. Of course, I want to acknowledge that in a large class, it can be difficult to meet everyone's unique needs at the same time, which is exactly why some folks look to private yoga as a solution.

That's what I told her. "Yes, that is a huge reason people turn to private yoga! To get that individualized attention, so you can learn and feel supported. That's how I started as well, after trying yoga studios and then turning to private yoga. In fact, yoga originally was taught one-on-one, with one student and teacher."

I went on to explain that I incorporate holistic aspects of yoga when I work with my students. We cover and practice asana, pranayama, mudras, and meditation, and if students are interested (and ready), we will weave in philosophy from texts and go over Patanjali eight limbs of yoga. Yoga is a holistic practice and study where one practices contemplation and self-inquiry, so that is how I practice and teach it.

She abruptly cut me off. "Oh no, I'm not interested in any of the spiritual or breathing stuff! I only want to learn the physical yoga to fix my back."

I looked over at my altar, at the statue of Buddha, the picture of my grandmother, the portrait of Guru Nanak, and the painting of Durga Mata for strength for this conversation. My free hand came over my forehead, and I slightly shook my head. Of course, I knew that some people were interested in yoga only for the physical benefits, but to hear it so clearly stated with a disregard for subtler practices and the deeper goals made me feel exasperated. This dismissal of the roots and true intents and goals is doing a disservice to the practice but even more so to us, to the depths we could reach.

I took a cleansing breath, sat up taller, and replied, "Well, yoga is a spiritual practice, and the way that I practice and teach, I will incorporate that in or at least hold that for myself as a grounding anchor and truth. There are even deeper goals to asana, and if you're looking for someone to only focus on teaching you asana and feeling better physically, unfortunately, I don't think I am the teacher for you. However, there are many other teachers that do exactly that and even those that specialize in injury rehab. I can provide some recommendations if you would like."

In the short pause after I finished speaking and then from the change of her tone, I could tell she was taken aback and not pleased with my answer. I put the phone face down on my desk, stood up, and shook my body intensely to shake off the energy of the call. I walked over to my bedroom and sat on my bed. Why did that bother me so much? I felt emotions of frustration, anger, and ickiness in my physical body. At the same time, I also felt humor rising to the surface. This was a reminder that we cannot be a teacher to every person, nor should we try.

This interaction highlighted once again the attitude and perception people have about yoga: the idea that you can pick and choose parts and not care about the ultimate goal and truth. Yoga is a complete practice and path, and asana is only one part of it. Patanjali, the compiler of the Yoga Sutras, lists asana as one of eight limbs of yoga, and asana is mentioned in only three of the 196 total sutras! Patanjali spends little time elaborating on asana other than to say "*sthira-sukham āsanam*," meaning asana is a steady and comfortable posture.

I want to be clear that I come to this conversation as an asana teacher myself and as someone who regards asana practice as sacred and transformative. In the early days of my own practice, there were many years where I practiced asana daily, sometimes for two to three hours. I saw what an impact it had on my physical, mental, and spiritual health. Asana practice helped to deepen my relationship to my body in a compassionate and curious way. By putting my body into unfamiliar shapes and breathing deeply, I began to see how my body is a vehicle and home for healing. Asana strengthened my physical body, helped me connect to my breath, and showed me the beauty of movement—both structured and intuitive. It calmed my mind, gave me relief from anxiety, and connected me to my energetic and subtle body. I continue to practice on an almost daily basis.

There is nothing wrong with cultivating a strong, healthy body—this is one of the reasons I practice asana. In fact, we need strong bodies to sustain us so that we can live fully within them for a longer period of time. Asana is a way of giving back to the body, nurturing it so that the mind can also grow strong. The mind-body connection is key, and cultivating both allows us to function with resilience and clarity. I often think of it as training to be a warrior: we need both body and mind to be in harmony. Through my practice, I've cultivated a strong body and a peaceful mind, and I encourage my students to do the same.

There are some students with whom we primarily focus on asana, mudras, and pranayama because that is where they are in their practice and readiness. In our modern ways of being, many of us are sedentary, and asana is the medicine we need. However, I help these students understand that while physical strength and health benefits are valuable, there are deeper, subtler levels to asana and to yoga itself that go beyond the physical.

When did the part become the whole? This interaction further illustrates how yoga is perceived in the West—as a physical fitness modality, a sixty-minute fitness class, a cure and remedy for physical ailments. This idea begins and ends with the physical body. Rather, if we are to see yoga as therapy, we should also consider the whole person, including their mental and emotional state—this is where we can turn toward the Koshas, to take in the full expanse of someone's being. For yoga to go deep, not only does someone's physical and mental health improve; their nature, personality, and psychological and psychic framework also change. As Swami Muktibodhananda shared in the Hatha Yoga Pradipika, "You should not merely feel freedom from disease, but freedom from bondage and from the vagaries of the mind." Otherwise, yoga, a practice and path for seeking self-realization, is used as a weapon to forward the agenda of what types of bodies are accepted, celebrated, and highlighted.

How Mass Media and Digital Media Portray Yoga

You don't have to look too far to see images of white, cis, thin, young bodies doing advanced acrobatic poses. The people in these images are often championed as the poster children of yoga. This heavily promotes certain beauty standards as being the ideal—which has no bearing on how talented or skilled a yoga teacher is. This excludes our trans, queer, disabled, BIPOC, fat, and elderly kin.

For years, *Yoga Journal* has been criticized for its cover model choices, featuring only white, cis, able-bodied folks in advanced asana poses. In a two-year archival study of the magazine, not one South Asian person was on the cover, and less than 1 percent of the content contributors were South Asian.

It has been criticized for promoting products like diet pills and expensive yoga pants designed for only thin and affluent women and for using sexualized images of women to sell their products. However, *Yoga Journal* wasn't always this way. When it was started in 1975 by the California Yoga Teachers Association, it took a much more diverse, grassroots approach led by volunteers and passionate contributors and covered more aspects of yoga in a genuine desire to share and teach.

For example, an issue in 1987 highlighted two AIDS survivors, Louis Nassabey and Don Turner, with the title "Living with Aids." The 1994 issue covered teachers like Malidoma and Sobonfu Some'—spiritual leaders and writers from the Dagara community in Burkina Faso, West Africa—speaking on radical ritual. And the 1997 issue showcased Maya Tiwari, a world peace leader and international teacher of Ayurveda from India, in an article titled "Earth Wisdom: Maya Tiwari Reveals the Roots of Ayurveda." In these earlier issues, all these people on the cover are shown sitting or standing and smiling. And none of them are in tight-fitting spandex or "yoga leggings."

It is also interesting to note how the subtitle changed over the years. In the earlier issues from 1985 and 1987, the subtitle read, "The Magazine for Conscious Living." Then in 1994, there was a shift to "For Health and Conscious Living." By 2000, these subtitles had been dropped, and a vast shift in cover models and content—to one much less diverse—started to reveal itself.

In 1998, John Abbott, a former investment banker and yoga practitioner, bought the publication. Then in 2006, the magazine was bought by Active Interest Media . . . and this is the *Yoga Journal* we see today.

There was a shift to content focusing on the health and well-being of the physical body; photographs that increasingly featured thin, lithe, able-bodied people in complex poses; and ads for wellness retreats, weight loss supplements, and expensive activewear.

The August 2009 cover shows Nicki Doane, a thin, white, athletic-looking able-bodied American woman wearing a matching light blue athletic set, in Eka Pada Rajakapotasana (One-Legged King Pigeon Pose), which is not easily or readily accessible to many practitioners, including myself. It also highlights the content inside, like "The Science of Stretching" and "All about Abs: 9 Poses for Core Strength."

The August 2018 issue highlights another thin white yoga teacher—Kathryn Budig—in Utthita Hasta Padangusthasana (Extended Hand-to-Big-Toe Pose), another more difficult pose. This edition also promises the following content inside: "12 Poses for Flexible Hips and Hamstrings" and "Teachers: Why You Should Stop Giving This Cue."

"Racism is so implicit that you never even notice that it's a white girl on the cover every single time," says Amy Champ, a PhD scholar from the University of California, Davis, who wrote her dissertation on American yoga. "When you begin to ask yourself, 'What does yoga have to do with my community?', then you begin to question all these inequities."

Later, in the wake of the racial unrest, riots, and protests triggered by the brutal murder of George Floyd during his arrest by Minneapolis police officers on May 25, 2020, *Yoga Journal*, alongside many other organizations, finally shifted its perspective and started highlighting teachers of color on its covers. Still, these teachers were shown in yoga leggings and tight tops, in different asana poses, and with headlines around them like "7 Poses to Release Tight Hips" and "Get Comfortable with Inversions."

Progress? Perhaps a little. *Yoga Journal* is just one publication, but its evolution reflects the increasing emphasis in America on yoga as physical fitness.

Social media and the digital space are other arenas where the preoccupations of Western yoga practice are clearly visible. A search on YouTube for the most popular yoga channels shows dozens of thin, cis, fit, young, and attractive creators listed as "most relevant" on the platform. Each one of these channels focuses on asana and the physical benefits of practice.

In an NBC News article, Sean Feit Oakes, a yoga instructor and industry expert, said, "The algorithm favors certain qualities. White people who already had a following were the most likely to thrive over quarantine. So a brown-skinned person is going to have a hill to climb. . . . Sexiness goes far."

This reality continues the narrative that to practice or teach yoga, you need to be flexible, young, thin, white, cis, able-bodied, and attractive in the standard sense as deemed by popular media. It excludes certain groups of people who don't see themselves represented by race, age, gender, shape, ability, or even socioeconomic status.

It reminds me of my initial search for yoga in Los Angeles and feeling excluded by the coldness of the teachers and staff, the speed at which the asana was practiced, and the matching expensive outfits. Those experiences meant that for the next year, I stopped seeking yoga and stopped practicing. As I suspect sadly happens to too many people, that was at a time in my life when yoga in its fullest and deepest sense could have eased a lot of anxieties, depression, and suffering.

One of my students, Leah, who is Black, a gifted speaker, a death doula, and a yoga teacher, told me about one of the vinyasa yoga classes she attended before beginning work with me as my private client. She walked into the studio, took her spot on her mat, and could feel people in the class staring at her. She said she had come to expect this as a bigger-bodied Black woman but was surprised that more people were looking at her than usual. Throughout the class, the instructor kept singling her out, adjusting her in the asana poses, and assuming she didn't know what she was doing. Leah had spent years building a loving relationship with her body and did not appreciate being told she was doing the poses "wrong," nor was she asked if she wanted the adjustments or the one-on-one attention.

At the end of the class, as Leah was rolling up her mat, the instructor came over and recommended the Hatha class, saying that is a gentler class and might be better suited for her. Leah, at a loss for words, just nodded her head and raced out of the studio.

An aside here: in addition to body-shaming my student, this yoga instructor oversimplified Hatha Yoga to mean "gentle asana." That is incorrect. Hatha Yoga is a complete path and system of yoga that is so much more than the modern definition of it as gentle poses held for a longer period of time than in other asana forms. Hatha is a Sanskrit word (pronounced "huh-tuh") that translates to *force*, *willful*, or *the yoga of forceful exertion*—the exact opposite of gentle. Pulling from tantric ritual, Hatha uses bodily effort to move subtle energies up the spine, with the goal of dissolving the mind in meditation.

Back to Leah. When she reached out to me, wanting to work with me privately, her message read, "I would like to book a virtual session with the intention of unpacking racial trauma."

Oof.

Our time together was spent unpacking the layers of racism that are present not only in the yoga studio space but also in America in general. Over several sessions, we spoke about how these messages get internalized. How we begin to believe them. Leah was invited into meditations to explore where these messages were internalized into her body and into longer holding poses to allow that tension and stress to seep out.

Leah expressed gratitude for being guided into a Supported Pigeon Pose (Eka Pada Rajakapotasana), where she had ample time to breathe deeply and was invited to notice where these racist messages were being held in her physical body. Before this, she hadn't realized a yoga practice could mean spending the time connecting via conversation and then being guided into only one to three poses, with an abundance of time and props to really check in. It didn't have to look like a vinyasa class at a studio.

Leah shared how she would shrink herself down in these studio spaces, not wanting to be seen. Everything changed for her when she began to practice at home, found me to practice with over Zoom, and then created her own spaces for others to feel safe enough to practice.

We spoke at length about internalized fatphobia, a term used to describe the internalization of societal beliefs and biases about body size and weight. Folks who have internalized fatphobia may hold negative beliefs about their own body size and shape and may feel shame about their weight. They may also hold negative beliefs about other people who are perceived as overweight or obese and may engage in stereotyping, discrimination, or bullying based on weight.

Commercialized, commodified yoga reinforces internalized fatphobia. It does this by emphasizing thinness, which can lead to discrimination against people who do not fit this narrow beauty standard. In addition, some yoga studios and classes are marketed and catered primarily to people who are already thin and "fit," leading to a further lack of diversity in the yoga community.

This disregards the fact that all bodies can be fit in the sense of being healthy. Fitness or health doesn't correlate to thinness.

Leah shared: "Certain yoga studios I teach at still have messaging like, 'Practice yoga for weight loss,' and that really bothers me. Because here the yoga studio is promoting this message and then the students have this preconceived notion of what to expect. But then when they walk into the class, they see me—a fat Black woman and think, how is *she* going to teach me about weight loss? I'm not here to teach yoga as a workout regimen, and this puts me in an incredibly awkward position."

How is it that yoga, a practice that is meant to create freedom and liberation, ends up being co-opted by the dominant culture to ostracize people who are seeking that very same freedom and liberation? And oftentimes such people are already within a marginalized community or deemed different from what is socially acceptable by the dominant culture. Deemed less-than. This only serves to perpetuate oppression and marginalization—the very thing that yoga, as a holistic practice of self-acceptance, stands against.

These modern asana classes have sadly become the norm: yoga has become synonymous with movement, and asana has become "conscious movement." Over my eleven years of visiting yoga studios all over the US, I became accustomed to being in the minority as a person of color, to expecting thin, fit, cis white people in Lululemon and Alo Yoga clothing, and to practicing movement for the purpose of fitness and my physical health.

The Holistic Goals of Yoga

The Western mainstream view of yoga is that it is an exercise system for health and fitness. While improvements and transformation in physical and mental health are natural consequences of yoga asana, the goal of the practice as it was originally intended is much more far-reaching and expansive, with the capacity to help us realize the interconnected nature of our being.

Depending on which lineage or tradition of yoga you investigate, the more holistic goals include discovering the truth of who you really are beyond this body and mind. It invites us to question the labels and limitations that we place on ourselves, or that others or society impose upon us. In holistic yoga practice, we tap into our consciousness and access our innate inner state of peace, wisdom, and freedom. For other paths, it is about union and harmonizing ourselves with the universe, with nature. Union with God/Goddess. To have a greater sense of meaning for why we are in existence today and how to work with our suffering, to be of greater service. One thing that is common throughout is that yoga is a path of expanding our perspective and awareness to grow our compassion and empathy with ourselves and all beings.

Contrary to the popular idea of yoga, the practice is about creating harmony—not discord or dissatisfaction—between our body and mind. Patanjali Yoga Sutras and the eight-limbed path are all about the science of mind transformation. Our mind is the window through which we perceive the world, and if this window is clouded, skewed, or even a little blurry, that is how we will perceive the world. Yoga can help uncloud the window. The window of our mind can become clouded or skewed due to trauma, unconscious biases, limiting self-beliefs, misperceptions, or societal conditioning. William Blake said, "If the doors of perception were cleansed every thing would appear to man as it is, Infinite." Walking the path of self-realization has nothing to do with how your body looks, what type of athletic clothing you own, how much money you have in your bank account, or how physically flexible you are.

So, how have we gotten here—where we practice asana divorced from its ethical and wisdom foundations?

Short History of Modern Yoga

Modern mobility asanas have roots in the Hatha school of yoga, which originated in the ninth to eleventh centuries. Some notable teachers of this time include yogis and realized masters, Matsyendra Natha and Goraksha Nath. You might also recognize these names because of asana poses like Matsyendrasana and Gorakshasana, which are named in honor of these enlightened beings. The Hatha path of yoga is a rich philosophical-spiritual system designed with a specific goal of reaching self-realization through meditation (dhyana). It presents a comprehensive roadmap, beginning with straightforward physical purifications (shatkriya) and asanas and then progressing to pranayama and intricate psycho-energetic adjustments (mudra and bandha), ultimately culminating in the achievement of self-realization through dhyana samadhi (meditative absorption). Hatha Yoga has its own established lineage, philosophies, perspectives on the cosmos, intricate knowledge of subtle physiology, meditation practices, rituals, symbolic representations, and ethical guidelines.

Hatha yogis moved the body into specific postures to impact the subtle body, which is composed of nadis (channels) through which prana (energetic life force) flows, to create suppleness in the limbs and prepare the body for further subtle practices like pranayama and meditation. Asanas were practiced for stability of the body and for mental calmness. By working with the prana, Hatha yogis stabilized the body to ready the mind for meditation and the ultimate goal of samadhi. **The focus is on developing stability in the body to refine both the energy and mind, not just for the purposes of stretching.** Hatha yogis knew that we should respect our body, as it is a way to go deeper within.

Imagine your body has two main energy channels, like rivers flowing in opposite directions. One channel, known as ida, is associated with the moon (calming energy, parasympathetic activation) and the other, known as pingala, is associated with the sun (active energy, sympathetic activation). Hatha Yoga aims to bring harmony to these twofold energies in the body. When the left nostril is open and breath is easefully flowing, it means ida is active, while if the right nostril is open and breath is easefully flowing, pingala is active. When the ida and pingala energies are balanced, they flow smoothly through a central channel called the sushumna, which flows along the spine from the mooladhara or root chakra (pronounced "chuk-ra") to the ajna or third eye chakra. This is like opening a clear pathway for your spiritual energy to rise. So, Hatha Yoga is the process of uniting "ha," the sun or pingala nadi, and "tha," the moon or ida nadi, with sushumna (the central channel for spiritual ascension) in the ajna chakra. Before the union can take place, there must be purification of all the body elements through practices like shatkriyas, asana, pranayama, and mudras.

Thus, it is important to have body purification practices like asana and the Hatha Yoga Pradipika, a classic fifteenth-century Sanskrit manual on Hatha yoga composed by Svatmarama, which emphasizes that practitioners begin with asana. "Since asana is the first part of hatha yoga, it is described first. One should practice asanas, which give stability, health, and lightness of limbs" (Hatha Pradipika 1.17). This text speaks of eighty-four asanas taught by Lord Shiva (who is supreme cosmic consciousness), from which it outlines the best fifteen, almost half of them involving dynamic actions such as bending, twisting, and balancing. Before this, yogic texts only spoke of asana as a way to sit (the definition of asana).

This is asana done with intention and the end goal of moving toward meditation and samadhi. Patanjali works with the mind and Hatha yoga works with the ways of prana to work on the mind. Both are working on the same thing—the mind—and are using different paths to get to the ultimate goal of samadhi.

However, there are certain Hatha practices that would be entirely unrecognizable today. The earliest postures of yoga included ascetics standing on one leg or holding an arm above their head for years. These are practices known as tapas to still the mind and burn away past karma.

During British colonist rule in the twentieth century, Hatha yoga practices were considered barbaric and practitioners were regarded as charlatans and masochists by British colonial officers, which influenced Indian elites to view them in a similar way. Poor Hatha yogis were forced to settle into urban areas, where they resorted to postural yogic showmanship and spectacle to earn money. Even Swami Vivekananda (1863–1902), who spoke at the 1893 Parliament of the World's Religions Fair in Chicago as a representative of Hinduism and India, having internalized this criticism, distanced himself from Hatha yoga and disparaged it.

The Reclamation of Yoga in India

Toward the end of colonial rule, Indians reclaimed physical yoga as a tool for self-empowerment. However, this reclamation wasn't entirely free from the influence of Western priorities such as the growing emphasis on physical fitness and validation by science. Indian teachers like Swami Kuvalayananda, Sri Yogendra, Sri Tirumalai Krishnamacharya, Swami Sivananda, K. Pattabhi Jois, T. K. V. Desikachar, and B. K. S. Iyengar revived the Hatha Yoga path in novel ways after the British deemed it "savage" and unacceptable for people to practice. In different ways, each one helped to revive the practice of asana, emphasized the health benefits of posture practice, developed yoga as exercise and therapy, and outlined systemic articulation of each asana.

Swami Kuvalayananda (1883–1966) sought scientific explanations for the various effects of yoga, and in 1924 he founded the Kaivalyadhama Health and Yoga Research Center in Lonavala to provide a laboratory for his scientific study of Yoga. He also started the first scientific journal devoted to scientific investigation into yoga, *Yoga Mimamsa*. Kuvalayananda devised the asana sequence of headstand, shoulder stand, prone backbends, seated forward fold, twisting poses, and arm balances. Later, Swami Sivananda would develop his own asana sequence inspired by Kuvalayananda's teachings.

Sri Yogendra (1897–1989) was the first yoga teacher to offer public classes with no selection process and with clear fees. In 1918, he taught the first public yoga course at a time when yoga was taught one-on-one between a guru and a student. He suited asana to meet a more modern audience wishing for health and recreation and taught dynamic sequences. Both Swami Kuvalayananda and Sri Yogendra had the same guru, Swami Madvadavasaji (1798–1921), who used yoga to treat the sick.

These two, alongside Tirumalai Krishnamacharya (1888–1989), made the physical methods of yoga more appealing in the twentieth century. It would be hard to find a modern asana tradition that Tirumalai Krishnamacharya, known as the father of modern yoga and from a lineage of the traditional Sri Vaishnavism, hasn't influenced. He was hired by the Maharaja of Mysore in the 1930s to spread yoga, and most of his students were young boys between twelve and eighteen.

The Maharaja of Mysore, a strong advocate for Indian independence, embraced yoga to cultivate strong youth. Krishnamacharya's employment and the emphasis on public yoga demonstrations stemmed from this vision. Krishnamacharya regularly utilized and taught the methodology of vinyasa krama.

However, when he taught vinyasa krama, it was not the vinyasa we see today, which we take to understand as a "flow yoga" class, or the sequence of chaturanga to upward dog to downward dog, which is overly simplified. The prefix *vi* means "in a special way" and *nyasa* means "to place." Thus, vinyasa actually means to *place in a special way* or to *intentionally arrange or link*. Vinyasa krama teaches us how to structure yoga asana practice intellectually—that it's not sufficient to merely take a step, but that that step must lead us in the correct direction and be executed in the appropriate manner. A practical example is being clear about which asana poses you want to do and knowing how to get ready for them to avoid any unwanted side effects. For example, Is your neck strong enough for a headstand? If your student is pregnant, what is appropriate to include and exclude? Being intelligent in your practice involves understanding the full picture of what you want to do and what your goal is, whether it's asana or pranayama, and getting ready for it by making necessary preparations and adaptations.

In Desikachar's book *The Heart of Yoga*, he is asked how his father Krishnamacharya saw the significance of asanas in the practice of yoga.

Desikachar responds,

> *My father never saw yoga simply as a physical practice. Yoga was much more about reaching the highest, which for him was God. . . . This path demands much more from those who follow it: a strong will, trust, and the ability to keep one's efforts constantly. . . . The steps in yoga that are concerned with the physical body are steps that should enable us to go the whole way, not the other way around. It is not a matter of*

> *making the body the center of all activities, nor of depriving it altogether. . . . Yoga is primarily a practice intended to make someone wiser, more able to understand things than they were before. If asanas help in this, terrific! If not then some other means can be found instead. The goal is always bhakti or, to put it in my father's words, to approach the highest intelligence, namely, God.*

Krishnamacharya was also one of the first to interpret the Yoga Sutras of Patanjali so that anyone could study them and have access to these teachings regardless of their belief system.

He was the teacher of his son T. K. V. Desikachar, of K. Pattabhi Jois, B. K. S. Iyengar (although it is said Iyengar did not spend much time under Krishnamacharya's tutelage), and Eugenie Peterson (who renamed herself Indra Devi), who all played a huge role in popularizing yoga asana in the West. Krishnamacharya played a role in creating the Ashtanga, vinyasa, and Viniyoga styles of yoga; his student Pattabhi Jois taught the Ashtanga vinyasa system; while his son T.K.V. Desikachar continued the legacy of Viniyoga and yoga therapy.

Perhaps it is both Pattabhi Jois (1915–2009) and Iyengar (1918–2014) who made the biggest impact on how asana is emphasized in modern-day practice. Pattabhi Jois taught the Ashtanga vinyasa system, where students learned fixed sequences of poses and added more on as they advanced. This is commonly what we see in modern yoga classes, where poses flow from one to the next. Jois produced hundreds of teachers through his teacher trainings, including my first teacher trainer for the 350-hour YTT I did in Australia. To help students understand how to get into postures, adjustments were offered by teachers, and some adjustments caused injury while others were inappropriate sexual touches. In 2019, Jois's grandson, R. Sharath Jois, who still leads world-wide asana tours, apologized for his grandfather's abuse.

B. K. S. Iyengar selected from Krishnamacharya's teachings to create Iyengar Yoga, which prescribed a disciplined form of body maintenance focused on alignment, biomechanics, and physical fitness as practice, referring to the body as a temple. He wrote, "To the yogi his body is the prime instrument of attainment. If his vehicle breaks down, the traveler cannot go far. If the body is broken by ill-health, the aspirant can achieve little." He used props like belts, bricks, and ropes to help the practitioner "conquer" the body. After publishing *Light on Yoga* (1966), which gave detailed instructions for poses and their benefits, he began training teachers in London—however, there was a condition for this to be funded by the government. Classes had to be presented as a workout—"provided that instruction is confined to 'asanas' and 'pranayamas' and does not extend to the philosophy of Yoga as a whole." Iyengar consented to this.

In 1948, Peterson opened a yoga studio in Hollywood, the first in Los Angeles, and taught many celebrity pupils. She taught yoga as exercise, left out the spiritual aspects, and catered to a white and wealthy clientele. She is often regarded as the "First Lady of Yoga," which disregards all the women who practiced and studied yoga before her in South Asia. I encourage people to read *Original Godmothers of Yoga* by Tejal Patel, host of the podcast *Yoga Is Dead*, to learn about influential South Asian yoginis.

In *From Here Flows the River: The Life and Teachings of Krishnamacharya*, written by A.G. Mohan, a student of Krishnamacharya's for eighteen years, Mohan reflected on how Krishnamacharya expressed sadness over the decline of a genuine dedication to the deeper aspects of yoga:

> *In one class, when discussing the Yoga Sutra, Krishnamacharya noted that punaranveshana (literally, 'to re-search,' or 'to search once more') was needed now. He felt the ancient practices that had declined over time needed to be explored once more and their value brought out. "Subjects are of two*

> *categories," he said. "One category can be learned merely through words, by listening and understanding—these are theoretical subjects, like the rules and analysis of grammar. The other category needs to be practiced, like music, cooking, martial arts, and yoga as well. Nowadays, the practice of yoga stops with just asanas. Very few even attempt dharana and dhyana [deeper meditation] with seriousness. There is a need to search once more and reestablish the practice and value of yoga in modern times."*

This is one big way the colonized take on the views of the colonizers. Under British colonial rule, people in the Indian subcontinent had to struggle with an internalized inferiority complex. This belief that yoga being taught in the traditional way would not be accepted or celebrated meant these teachers changed their teachings, adapting to the expectations of the dominant culture. This is a long-term consequence of colonialism. This inferiority complex still rears its ugly head today.

Confirming to Dominant Culture

In one of our sessions, Leah shared with me how she began teaching at a local yoga studio in Maryland that hired her because they wanted to teach "authentic yoga" and teach more of the eight limbs of yoga. However, she soon started to get texts from the owner, telling her not to use mantras or Sanskrit in class because it was alienating the students.

Leah told me, "These yoga studios are picking up on the buzzwords floating around the industry and using those on purpose to make themselves seem inclusive and diverse. In reality, the studios screaming the loudest about being authentic are causing the most harm. I had thought that maybe this is a studio where I would be accepted, because it gave that impression of diversity, but it was not the case. Once I started teaching, I was told to stop chanting 'om' in class and using Sanskrit names for the poses. Once again, I came into a situation where a studio's actions did not match their words and I felt unsafe."

I can see why Indian yoga teachers felt they needed to strip certain aspects away for the Western audience—they must have experienced a similar level of misunderstanding and insistence on forsaking the authenticity of the teachings in the superficial attempt to make them more acceptable. This is not the yoga that saved my life and made me feel like I belong—in this world, in my body, and in relationship to myself and others.

That yoga encompasses the depth of the teachings. And that yoga doesn't require our bodies to look a certain way. This yoga, true yoga, is for all bodies, shapes, and sizes.

My Short-Lived Time Teaching at Yoga Studios

When I started teaching yoga in 2018, I taught only at a yoga studio for the first six months and then quickly left. I did not feel safe or comfortable teaching in modern yoga studios where the message of yoga is diluted to equate it with exercise for fitness's sake, and I was also the only person of color on the teaching staff. Oftentimes, I felt like a token hire, hired to show that the studio was "authentic" and "diverse."

I was teaching at a yoga studio in New Orleans, and as I was getting set up at the front of the class, putting down my yoga mat, and feeling obliged to connect my phone to the overhead speakers to play music, a student I had not met before walked up to me.

"Hi, good to meet you! The teacher that used to teach this class always kicked our butts, and I loved that workout. Do you think today we could focus on toning our butts?"

She turned sideways, wagged her butt, and winked at me, a big smile on her face, like we were now conspiring together. Momentarily stunned, I replied, "I'll see what I can do!"

Satisfied, she patted my arm and made her way back to her mat.

Turning away, I internally laughed while thinking with some terror, How will I be able to please this student?!

The way yoga is sold and marketed positions the teachers as service providers, where we feel compelled to please our students, the customers. Even if that comes at the cost of our ethics. I felt that weight on me from the studio owners, who paid us extra for the number of students in each class. If students had the perception that yoga is a workout, I, as a teacher, felt the need to make them feel like they got their money's worth.

This pressure was not for me. Soon, I stopped teaching at studios altogether. I didn't want to feed this narrative. As I have continued as a yoga teacher, I have given a lot of thought to what I'd like to offer. My own teachers have talked about the importance of finding clarity on what yoga is *for me* and anchoring into that.

Perception of the Body Over Time by Varying Yogic Traditions

Yoga Sutra 2.5 reads "*anityāśuci-duḥkhānātmasu nitya-śuci-sukhātma-khyātir avidyā*." The translation is "Ignorance is the notion that takes the self, which is joyful, pure, and eternal, to be the nonself, which is painful, unclean, and temporary."

Here Patanjali gives a very important definition of ignorance, the primary cause of all mental bondage: ignorance (avidya) is confusing the nature of the soul with that of the body. The body is described as painful (dukkha), unclean (ashuci), and temporary (anitya), while the true self or soul (purusha) is joyful (sukha), pure (shuci), and eternal (nitya).

Edwin F. Bryant translates the above sutra as, "Although one may think that one's body, one's mind, and even one's possessions are one's real self, they are not, and to confound them as such is ignorance." Vyasa is the first translator and commentator of the

Yoga Sutras in the fifth century CE, and as Bryant illustrated in his commentary on the Yoga Sutras of Patanjali, "It cannot be overstated that Yoga philosophy is Patanjali's philosophy as understood and articulated by Vyāsa."

Vyasa, also known as Vedavyasa or Vyasadeva, is considered the "sage of sages" and the primary literary figure of ancient India. He is regarded as the author of the Mahabharata and the Puranas and is also known for dividing the Vedas into four parts—*Rig Veda, Sama Veda, Yajur Veda*, and *Atharva Veda*—making them easier to study and understand.

There are various views of the body in dharmic knowledge systems. Tantra considers the body to be a divine vessel, bhakti sees the body as a tool that can be used in the service of God/Goddess, Ayurveda views it as a complex biological system requiring balance, and The Karma Sutra (desire texts) focus on the body's potential for pleasure.

These viewpoints are not mutually exclusive but coexist within the broader framework. In contrast, ascetic traditions often hold a more critical view, considering the body as a temporary and imperfect vessel, emphasizing its limitations and impermanence. No matter how beautiful the body, at the end of the day, it is a bag of bodily fluids and organs. For example, Buddha advised his followers to contemplate the reality of the impurities of the body. For centuries, these ascetics and forest-dwelling yogis—even before the Buddha's time (around 500 BCE) and continuing long after Patanjali (around 200 CE)—believed that to break free from the cycle of rebirth, they needed to transcend their physical bodies. Tantra, which began around the fourth to sixth centuries CE, brought a revolutionary idea: if everything is ultimately divine Spirit, then our bodies are not something to be overcome but sacred expressions of that very Spirit. Tantric practitioners aimed to transform and worship the body as a way to unite with the divine. These tantric rituals, including purifying ways to manipulate breath and other vital energies, chanting mantras, and visualizing subtle phenomena, were combined with ascetic objectives to then later shape Hatha Yoga. Hatha yogis spoke about respecting the body to go deeper within.

In short, *most* yogic traditions view the physical body as a temporary vessel and not the ultimate source of happiness or enlightenment. The body is temporary and always changing. There is a clear call here to seek joy in what is eternal, which is the soul and not the material world. A true practice of yoga allows us to experience the radical truth that we are all worthy and born divine. We are already whole and complete because we are pure consciousness. As my teacher Sri Prasad Rangnekar says, "I am eternal True Self experiencing myself and the world through this body, mind, and life."

A holistic practice of yoga can help us to feel more at home in our bodies, to accept our bodies, to know that they will change with time and age, and to accept and love and welcome all bodies. This allows us to accept the nature of reality around our bodies as always changing, which can be quite opposite to our modern society obsessed with retaining youth in any way possible. It can also teach us that we are more than our bodies, that we are divine consciousness, and that peace and well-being are always available to us. I think that's so much better than simplifying yoga to be exercise for the toning of our physical body.

4

THE MANY PATHS (MARGAS) OF YOGA

Asana Practiced with Intent and Pratyahara

YOGA REMINDS US of our sovereignty and personal power to make choices and align ourselves in ethical and moral ways for the betterment of all beings. Our personal freedom is tied to collective liberation. I turn to this quote generally attributed to philosopher Jiddu Krishnamurti: "It is no measure of health to be well adjusted to a profoundly sick society." To be truly well is to acknowledge and cultivate a transpersonal state of harmony, where mutual respect and care is extended to everything you are in relationship with.

Entering states of relaxation might be a side effect of practice but was never meant to be the ultimate goal. Through the stillness, silence, and sensory withdrawal of pratyahara (fifth limb on Patanjali's eightfold path), and one-pointed concentration, we seek to still the mind so that we really know ourselves—and in turn the nature of consciousness and the world. In knowing ourselves, we can free ourselves, know the roots of suffering, and then work to free everybody else. Asana is shared as a tool to steady the mind, not the end goal in itself.

However, the asana classes I have been part of have included loud, bumping music, mirrors all around, and too many people squeezed into a small room—these factors present abundant sensory distractions. This, to me, does not create the proper conditions for the mind to focus on the practice and find steadiness. Loud music can distract rather than focus. The mirrors mean you might be focusing on what your physical body looks like, bringing attention outside of yourself. Consciously or unconsciously, being in a room with that many people might encourage students to compare their practice with others. To compete with the person next to them.

This comparison and competitiveness results in the mind losing its steadiness. Instead of going within, the attention travels outside. Yoga is not meant to be about being perfect in comparison to others. This, in my view, causes a great deal of harm. Lots of modern yoga classes don't encourage inward focus but instead emphasize the importance of outward focus on perfect postures.

Asana is not about perfecting postures or attaining the perfect shape. They're a way to explore and understand how our bodies move and function. In the long run, the focus isn't on mastering any particular pose but on utilizing these explorations to cultivate greater strength, skill, and a deeper connection with our physical intelligence. Ultimately, asana aims to empower us to use our bodies with intention and awareness, allowing us to be fully present in the moment. We learn how to live more comfortably and skillfully in our body.

Asana practice is one wonderful way to move from awareness of gross (large, obvious) sensations to smaller and subtler ones. An example of this comes from a student I worked with for three months on a weekly basis. When I would ask him to observe his body and mind and share what he was feeling the first few times we met, he would say something like "My lower back hurts and I feel tired." Then, slowly over time, he began to notice the breeze on his skin, the feel of his body in connection with the ground. He was able to describe in more detail how he was feeling beyond just tired.

This is interoception, the ability to sense internal signals from the body, like knowing when you are hungry or thirsty, hot or cold, or being able to sense the speed of your heartbeat or the feel of your breath. Interoception is important for us to be able to self-regulate and know what is going on. There have been more than a few times where I pondered why I felt *so anxious* and began to spiral, thinking I needed to drastically change something about my life. Then when I really checked in with myself, I realized the dull ache in my stomach wasn't due to anxiety but hunger! We need to be able to check in with ourselves to take care of ourselves and our biological needs. Otherwise, we are liable to make mountains out of molehills.

I encourage my students to spend at least thirty minutes of every day in silence. No phone, music, TV, books, or podcasts. This time can be spent seated or lying outdoors, listening to the birds and sounds of nature. I often do this myself, to ask what wisdom and medicine nature holds for me on any given day. Using this skill of deep listening, I have received messages from my body and nature. You might choose to spend this time meditating, whether seated or walking, or making something with your hands. I have called this time my scheduled "boredom time" or my deep listening time. Learn to tune in to the natural world around you. Since 2018, I have dedicated sixty-eight days to complete silence during Vipassana Meditation retreats. These extended periods of deep meditation have been profoundly clarifying and revealing, offering insights that continue to shape my understanding and awareness.

The poem "A Great Yogi" by Sant Mirabai inspires me to return to silence to tune in. Mirabai is a celebrated Bhakti saint, known for her devotional poetry and love for Krishna.

In my travels I spent time with a great yogi.
Once he said to me.
"Become so still you hear the blood flowing
through your veins."
One night as I sat in quiet,
I seemed on the verge of entering a world inside so vast
I know it is the source of
all of
us.

True realized teachers of yoga taught that yoga brings us to self-authority. To trust in ourselves and our inner wisdom, not to outsource to external sources. Yoga teaches us about the importance of silence and going within, to the source of all that exists. Asana's function for classical yoga is to train the body so that it does not disturb or distract the mind of the yogi in any way when sitting in meditation.

So how can we practice asana in a yogic way? The objectives of practice matter here—an asana class needs to be presented in a way for students **to be more concentrated** and find ways to keep their attention anchored. This reduces the possibility of distraction and a wandering or comparing mind.

Asana shouldn't be practiced in any old way. Beer yoga and goat yoga are bewildering to me. How can you focus when a goat is pooping on your mat? And how can you find clarity if your mind is being clouded by alcohol?

I offer these suggestions:

1. Set an intention, or sankalpa, for your practice. Greater awareness begins with intention. Why am I practicing or teaching? What's the *why* here? An intention can give the busy mind a place on which to anchor as we move through the movement. And so what should the intention be?

   Us contemporary yoga practitioners tend to associate the English word *intention* with a goal. In Sanskrit, intention is sankalpa. Sankalpa is less about goal setting, about asking what we can get, and more about asking, What do I promise to bring? Sankalpa is not a goal but a commitment. Your sankalpa is where you'll rest your active mind.
2. Observe everything. Observe your sensations, reactions, wandering mind, and so on, without criticism and judgment. Yoga is about increasing self-knowledge. Notice what your mind and body are doing while practicing asana. Keep bringing your focus on yourself and your practice.
3. Practice dharana or one-pointed concentration. During practice, have an anchor for your mind to be able to find

steadiness and absorption without distraction. Focus on your breath, focus on what is going on in your body, or focus on where your gaze (drishti) is. Commit to noticing the breath. Commit to witnessing your movement without aversion. Commit to staying present. You get to choose.

4. To reduce outside distractions, try practicing without music.
5. Practice slowly. There is no rush or sense of urgency that is needed in practice.
6. Practice ahimsa, or nonharm. Be gentle and kind with yourself during practice. It does not matter if you can hit perfect alignment in posture or place your leg behind your head or if the student next to you appears "more advanced." This also reduces the likelihood of injury! I have often seen students pushing themselves in asana practice, neglecting this principle of ahimsa, and violating their own boundaries.

On Paths of Yoga versus Styles of Asana

To continue the discussion of asana and how it fits into the holistic practice of yoga, it's necessary to dig into the many different paths of yoga and how they do or don't relate to the different schools of yoga practice that are commonly presented in the West.

After telling people that I am a yoga teacher or yoga student, more times than not, I am then asked the question, "Oh, what style of yoga do you teach or practice?"

I struggle with this because when people are asking this, they are really asking, What style of asana do you teach or practice? How fast or slow? Is it heated? Is it vinyasa, gentle, Ashtanga, restorative, Power, yin?

Styles of asana have really become popular over just the last sixty years as various teachers and schools have created their own systems and sequences.

What has also become common in modern or popular yoga is branded asana styles: Bikram, CorePower, vinyasa, Iyengar, Baptiste, Rocket, Power yoga, et cetera. This can happen when a popular teacher has created their own brand of yoga, most often including only asana, and gone to market with that. They wanted to create their own identities (brands) through their own ways of practice and teaching. No wonder students are confused!

One of these branded styles of yoga that I have some personal experience in is Baptiste yoga. I took a training in Baptiste yoga shortly after I moved to New Orleans. I didn't know many people in New Orleans, and I didn't have any yoga connections either. So I took to the internet, searching for yoga jobs and local studios. I came across an opening teaching Baptiste yoga. It was not something I had heard of before, but I was intrigued. In order to teach Baptiste yoga, I first had to be trained in it.

At the training, I had no idea what to expect. The women at the front desk welcomed me in with a smile and pointed me down a hallway to the room we were all going to be in. I took my sandals off and gingerly walked into the room. It was well lit, with white walls and brown wood floors—an aesthetic I had grown accustomed to in the yoga studio world. As the room filled up and we got started, I observed that I was the only brown person in the room, surrounded by white cis people in tight spandex clothing. By this point, I had come to accept this as the norm and merely noted it as another class that held the same narrative in the modern yoga space. I also became used to becoming a chameleon in these spaces, using my shared identities of privilege of able-bodiedness, thinness, light skin, being cis, and shared language to camouflage and fit in. The lead trainers were two charismatic and tall people who had studied for years with Baron Baptiste—the "pioneer" of this yoga method.

We got started learning the Journey into Power Sequence, a vinyasa yoga sequence or "methodology" that Baptiste had created, where specific poses flowed into one another without any breaks or holds. This was a faster-paced asana practice, where breath had to be controlled to move from one pose to another without stopping.

I found this interesting, especially much later. This creating and founding of brands and styles of yoga, where the founder has put together a specific sequence of poses and labeled it as their own. This plethora of yoga styles can come from consumeristic desires—to allow the teacher to portray themselves as different or unique as opposed to their competition, so that they attain more students to their brand, sell more branded yoga mats, enroll more yoga teacher trainees in their "specific style of school," sell more retreats, and the list goes on. Consumerism seems to have no end point. As the Bhagavad Gita reminds us, desire is never satiated and burns like fire (3.39).

At the same time, I know students and teachers going into the path of yoga are typically sincere and considerate folks who know that when we practice and teach, we receive so much. Is it that capitalism pulls everything into its wake? I struggle with this myself as a yoga teacher, finding that balance of returning to yoga's roots and creating space for innovation, selling our services as many of us do, whether private yoga teachers, studio teachers, or course leaders. The line I draw for myself is, in my work, am I losing my own integrity or yoga's integrity to make money? Am I causing harm to myself or others or exploiting others or this land to make money?

Bikram Choudhury did something very similar when he put twenty-six poses together and branded it Bikram yoga. He even went as far as trying to trademark the sequences of poses in 2011, which thankfully failed. Trying to trademark or own parts of yoga speaks to a colonial mentality to me, where ownership needs to be staked. This path and practice are meant for all to understand, and to embody with respect and time. Not to be stripped down, renamed, and rebranded. Does anyone own yoga? I don't think so. Instead, we endeavor to study and practice with respect. To honor this thousands-year-old tradition. To learn from and uplift the original stewards of this ancestral practice.

At the end of the first day of the Baptiste training, I walked over to the lead trainer and expressed my resistance to moving so quickly and having to follow the alignment so closely. I felt that it wasn't an accessible sequence for many folks. She enthusiastically clapped and said, "Resistance is great! Keep powering through! Through resistance is the breakthrough. Remember—be a yes."

Being a yes was something I heard several times throughout the first day. It was taught as an internal commitment to being there and committing to the program and to your transformation. That nothing would change if students didn't wholeheartedly want to be there and had resistance, fear, cynicism, or resignation.

This messaging—say yes, be here, be committed, don't have any worries, trust me, don't think so hard, just feel—smacks of cultlike thinking and new age spirituality to me.

Critical Thinking in Yoga: Yes, Judgment Is Okay

Yoga is all about critical thinking and using our discernment (viveka). To blindly believe and trust in someone because they say so is not using our critical thinking skills. Patanjali even points to this in Yoga Sutra 2.26: "The means to liberation is uninterrupted discriminative discernment." It's crucial and healthy to have doubt. It's important to learn to discern and distinguish one thing from another. This creates room for us to see things clearly and ask for more clarity if it's not making sense or causing confusion.

In yogic philosophy, the term *viveka* refers to the faculty of discrimination or discernment between what is real and what is temporary or illusory. Viveka is an essential aspect of the yogic path, as it enables practitioners to navigate through the complexities of life and spiritual growth. It involves cultivating clarity, wisdom, and a deep understanding of the true nature of reality. Viveka helps individuals make wise and ethical choices in life. It allows one to discern between actions that contribute to personal growth, well-being, and spiritual evolution and actions that lead to suffering, attachment, and ignorance. By exercising viveka, individuals align their actions with higher values, ethical principles, and their inner truth.

I think of the commonly shared story in yogic and Buddhist teachings of the person stumbling upon a snake on their path and becoming quite frightened, only to realize it was a rope all along. Had the person not investigated using light, they would have continued on in their ignorance, full of fear. What is needed is clear sight, to investigate and realize that we are often mistaken, we cannot always believe what we perceive.

Viveka to me is the understanding that you must tune into the teacher within, the wisdom and truth within. *Yoga is an experiential system of spirituality. It is not dogma. Doubt is healthy and discernment is required and encouraged on this path.*

I didn't ultimately buy into the Kool-Aid of Baptiste yoga. Mainly because I didn't have the thousands of dollars to invest in the training, and I felt an uneasiness with the lack of history, philosophy, and acknowledgment of the roots of yoga.

Baron Baptiste, Brian Kest (who created Power yoga), and Larry Schultz (who created TM Rocket) all serve as examples of white American men who went to India in their twenties to study with Indian teachers such as K. Pattabhi Jois and B. K. S. Iyengar and who came back to the US to create their own brands. All three of their brands focus on asana as the primary teaching and practice, asana that is more fast-moving and rigorous. *Power yoga* is a generic term primarily used to describe a vigorous vinyasa class. I'm sure these men started out passionate about yoga and its benefits and most likely had pure intentions. However, I am interested in the lasting impact.

This represents what is commonly found in modern yoga brands. People creating their own brands of yoga and systematizing things in their own way. Along the way, things are distorted, diluted, and completely changed. I think about the telephone game here. By the time it gets to the last person, the words are completely different! I often find myself conflicted: Yoga has continuously evolved with the times and is not static. However, how far are some of these modern yoga brands moving away from the original intentions and goals? I think it is our duty as yoga teachers and students to have healthy doubt and seek to see more clearly so that what we teach is not distorted.

***

The Different Paths of Yoga

It takes a lot of maturity to acknowledge the debts we owe to those who give and pass down knowledge. None of us are self-made, as much as the American dream wants to convince us of this.

In traditional yoga, the student–teacher relationship is an integral part of the path. This is referred to as the guru–shishya parampara. The traditional pedagogy of yoga is based on knowledge and wisdom transfer from the teacher (the acharya or guru) to the student, and this also includes directing the student experientially so that the teachings become embodied and not just understood intellectually. Yoga is meant to be lived and applied throughout life, and having a teacher helps with that guidance. A teacher can show you the path, and then it is your responsibility to walk on that path, to experiment and reflect. A good teacher is also able to compassionately hold a mirror up to us, to show us where further refinement is needed. This relationship is one of intimacy and trust. Education, in this way, is more than just sharing knowledge; it's about cultivating experiential wisdom and encouraging contemplative inquiry. This is something I think we are losing in how modern yoga is shared.

Students have expressed to me how lacking they found their yoga teacher trainings, and a part of that was the teacher–student relationship. With ten to forty people—or more—in a training, you are not getting the intimate relationship that was found in traditional times. You lose out on the mentorship and support that is so needed on this path. I've had to seek out one-on-one teachers myself, outside of the yoga teacher training context, and their support has helped me to be guided in the right direction. I think it is important to have a foundational understanding of yoga from a traditional perspective before we begin innovating ourselves or joining other schools of yoga, where perhaps anything might go.

We are highly indebted to the yogis of the past for their studies and acquired wisdom. We can turn to the paths, or margas of yoga here. Traditional yoga margas offer a complete system of philosophy and a set of practices that aim to move the student toward atma jnana (self-realization) and out of cycles of suffering to moksha (final liberation).

The four main paths, or margas, typically talked about are:

1. Bhakti: love and devotion
2. Jnana: knowledge
3. Raja: body and mind transformation
4. Karma: connected selfless service

These paths have their own unique practices and goals. And these are not the only ones! There are additional paths as well, such as Hatha Yoga, Laya yoga, Tantra yoga, and Nada yoga. The Bhagavad Gita mentions eighteen types of yoga as well. Let's break down each one of these paths.

Bhakti Yoga

Bhakti yoga emphasizes the cultivation of devotion, love, faith, and surrender to a personal deity, God/Goddess, a higher power, or the divine. It is considered the path of the heart, of developing humility and deep emotional connection and love for the divine. Practitioners express their devotion through chanting, performing kirtan, reciting prayers, offering puja (worship) to deities, and engaging in ceremonies. Deities commonly worshipped and revered include Sri Krishna, Lord Shiva, Durga Mata, Green Tara, and many more.

These deities can be invited into the home through statues, idols, pictures—otherwise known as murtis—and symbolic icons. You are inviting their living energy into your home, which is why you ensure their living area, say the altar, is kept clean and daily offerings are made. I sit in front of my altar every morning and pray and meditate. I always make sure to have water, flowers, a lit candle, incense, and/or fruits as offerings. I am always perplexed when I see yoga studios and other spaces that have statues and pictures just for decoration and the statue of Ganesh covered in dust! You wouldn't invite a friend over as a guest and then ignore them completely. Why would you do the same to a deity? Bhakti yoga teaches us to have reverence and to turn to deities as representations of the divine, where a spiritual relationship can be cultivated.

The ultimate goal of Bhakti yoga is to attain a complete union or absorption with the divine, known as bhava or prema. Bhakti is for the serious bhakta committed to intertwining their own being with that of their ideal—their ishta. This is where the translation of the word *yoga* as *to yoke* or *to unite* comes true as a goal. Mirabai's life and story showcases what unwavering devotion and Bhakti look like—she cast off all social and familial expectations to be with her love, Krishna. It is said that Krishna granted her to merge with a statue of himself so she could finally become one with him.

Bhakti yoga practitioners emphasize the practice of selfless service (seva) and to serve others with love and compassion. There is an understanding that we are all interconnected beings, and by doing service, we acknowledge how this helps everybody in the process—including ourselves. Sikhism was influenced by the Bhakti movement, and I was raised to learn from teachings from Sikh gurus like Guru Nanak and Guru Gobind Singh. Within Sikhism, there is the concept of the sant-sipahi, the warrior-saint. The warrior who fights and stands up for justice. And the saint who is wise and loves.

As a form of devotion, my dad would also always chant, "Waheguru, Waheguru" throughout his day, whether mentally or out loud.

Waheguru is the Sikh word for God and is often understood to mean "Wondrous Teacher" or "Wow! to the teacher who dispels darkness." It is a way to address and praise the divine, acknowledging its infinite nature, beauty, and wisdom and to have that state of wonder. For Sikhis, uttering or chanting "Waheguru" serves as a form of meditation and a way to connect with the divine presence that is around us and within us.

This is not something I personally began practicing until the beginning of 2023, when my yoga teacher "prescribed" this mantra to me and said to constantly repeat it mentally. I have found it brings me great peace and shifts my attention and awareness from any anxiety and ruminating thoughts to this practice of japa meditation, which allows my mind to quiet down. In this way, I am also surrendering to the divine to say, I trust you and have faith. One of my friends was given a small prayer box that says, "Worry less, pray more" by her Christian mom, and this rings true in this case.

Love also means the courage to honestly look at yourself and the world around you and not maintain a status quo that causes harm.

Reflection question:

- In your life, is there any practice you already do to express your devotion and gratitude?
- Is there a particular deity, teacher, or ishta that brings you relief or inspires you?
- Is there an inspirational figure from your ancestral and cultural lineage you can learn about?
- Do you pray or have a gratitude journal?
- Is there a mantra, song, or prayer that helps you connect with your inner self or the divine? How does it influence your state of mind and heart?

I encourage students to have at least one daily practice that helps them connect to the feeling that there is something greater than them. For me, I get a feeling of awe and wonder when I hike up to the top of a mountain and look out, struck by the beauty of nature. How expansive this world is. I sense intimately that I am in the presence of something boundless and unlimited that transcends my current comprehension of the world. Nature, to me, is divinity in action.

Having faith and devotion in the divine on this path as a yoga student and teacher provides an anchor to return to throughout the change and chaos of life. What are you devoted to? What do you turn to when you need strength? I turn to the yogic teachings; I turn within; I turn to my living teachers; I turn to nature and finding awe in the world around; I turn to Buddha, Guru Nanak, Durga Mata and Saraswati Ma; and I turn to sangha, to spiritual community.

Jnana Yoga

Jnana yoga is the path of intellect and knowledge as a way to burn away avidya (ignorance) to gain self-knowledge. It is an intellectual approach to spiritual evolution with basis in scriptures such as the Vedas or Upanishads, as well as reason and experience. The sadhak, or spiritual practitioner, on this path studies what is written and then reasons whether it is correct by using real life experience to see if it is true. Thus, you are not working from blind faith.

The goal is to deeply understand oneself by reading scriptures and acquiring knowledge and then testing to see whether it is true through direct, lived experience. Take, for example, the Bhagavad Gita. Anyone can buy a copy and then theoretically have all the information and knowledge needed for self-realization and enlightenment. However, reading through the text doesn't equate to immediate self-realization. Instead, you have to deeply study it, read it multiple times, and even spend your whole lifetime applying the teachings to your life until you truly understand it and absorb it into your awareness.

I'm sure many people can relate to cramming for an important test and wishing learning through osmosis was possible! If only I could learn everything by simply putting my head against the textbook to allow it to seep into my brain. But it is only by spending time and diving deep that we truly learn. This is why we say yoga is a path that may take lifetime(s) to understand.

The yogic teaching of the niyama, santosha, teaches us to have contentment and gratitude for our present circumstances. As an example, while writing this book, I have caught myself feeling irritated and thinking, "This project would be better if I just had more time!" I noticed the discontentment arising within me, and I noticed where I could breathe into those places to create more space. I then used an affirmation such as, *I am doing the best I can with my current conditions, and that is enough*. This strongly eased my anxiety and allowed me to find acceptance. I also then felt gratitude that I had this project at all!

Thus, to practice Jnana yoga effectively, one must possess the patience to engage in repeated efforts over time, consistently building knowledge and self-awareness. Jnana yoga reminds me that we are all scientists, testing out theories in our lives. Jnana yoga is based on the belief that true understanding and enlightenment can be attained through the direct realization of one's own innate knowledge and the transcendent wisdom that underlies all existence.

Jnana yoga encourages seekers to question and investigate the nature of reality, the self, and ultimate truth. Exploring questions like:

- Who am I?
- What is the nature of reality?
- What is consciousness?
- What is the relationship between all three of these?
- Why do we suffer?
- What is the meaning of life? (I add this one for myself.)

We explore these questions to hopefully come to the realization, the freedom in recognizing, that we are not the limited beings we have taken ourselves to be. To understand that we are already whole and complete and that wholeness is within us. It doesn't waver, it is always there and will always be there.

One of my teachers, Charlotte Nguyen, led a group of BIPOC through a meditation. She shared with us, "Recognize the inherent dignity within you. Allow the crown of your head to reach up toward the sky. This dignity is something that can never be taken away; it is innate and something you are born with [we are all born with]. No situation or person can take this dignity away."

To understand this reality requires a whole yoga practice. It requires skills of deep reflexivity and introspection and of looking deep within at our experiences. For marginalized communities, oppressed communities, and those in the global majority, messages of not being good enough, of being less-than, and of needing to prove our worth are rampant. *Yoga reminds us that is not true.* We were born whole, and we will die whole. Any yoga practice, yoga brand, or yoga teacher that tells you any different is not practicing or teaching yoga, and I would recommend staying far away from anyone who makes you question your worth.

Jnana yoga emphasizes the faculty of discrimination (viveka) to distinguish between the permanent and the impermanent and vichara (right inquiry) to distinguish the real and the unreal. It involves discerning the illusory nature of the world and the limitations of the mind and senses in perceiving the ultimate truth.

Reflection question: Think about one belief that you hold about yourself. *I am smart, I am dumb, I am a good writer, I am not good at math,* et cetera. Where did this belief come from? Is it true? Now think of one belief that you used to hold about the world that ended up being untrue or wrong. Were you able to graciously admit you were wrong, or did it feel difficult? Take at least five to twenty minutes to journal on this.

Raja Yoga

Raja yoga is the path that focuses on harmonizing and controlling the mind to gain spiritual growth and self-realization. Raja means *royal, supreme*, or *kingly*, and we can understand this path to be one where we have ownership over our minds. You are the king or ruler of your mental world. Patanjali's eight limbs of yoga, Hatha Yoga, and Kundalini yoga all lead to Raja Yoga. The Hatha Yoga Pradipika lays out physical modalities like kriyas, asana, pranayama, mudra, and bandha as ways to work with the body to refine the mind. The mind is refined for the ultimate pursuit of samadhi—this process is Raja yoga. The Hatha Pradipika defines Raja Yoga as a pursuit of samadhi.

This path requires consistent practice on the body and the mind. By stilling the various kinds of thought waves, this leads to the unveiling of the yoga that we already are. This process leads to the dissolution of the body and the mind to reveal ourselves as pure consciousness.

This is not a path that says only work on the body for physical prowess or the mind for greater relaxation. It is a systematic way of working to refine the mind to realize how interconnected we all are. By transforming the self, we are also helping to transform society and the universe.

Reflection question: Sit comfortably in a quiet place and take a few breaths to steady yourself. With eyes closed, mentally repeat the affirmation of "I am"—notice whether your mind races to quickly fill in the sentence with such as "I am sad" or "I am frustrated." Now try it again and let there be space and quiet after the "I am." What do you notice now? In this practice, I tuned more into the sensations of my body and into my senses. One time, doing this practice outdoors, a bird chirped and I felt, "I am this bird."

Karma Yoga

Karma yoga is action. It is a path of selfless service and building of compassion to counteract the influences of egoism, the problem of "me-me-me." This path helps to purify the mind to recognize what self-centered tendencies you hold and to aspire to dedicate yourself to all life forms. True selfless action comes in taking actions without expectations of receiving anything in return. In the Bhagavad Gita, it is described as knowing we have the right to take action but not to expect a certain result, and any result we do receive is a gift from God/Goddess. Karma yoga helps us to realize we are not fully in control and to give up seeing ourselves as the center of the world.

In modern yoga, businesses and studios have co-opted Karma yoga and principles like seva to have people work for free. In exchange for services like cleaning the studio, managing the front desk, and teaching unpaid community classes, newer yoga teachers are given free classes at the studio. This is not Karma yoga—this is bartering. Businesses are taking advantage of spiritual concepts to help themselves advance. Karma yoga and seva are done when the individual chooses to take selfless actions to give back *without expecting anything in return.* When the student knows the action is being taken because we are all interconnected. When I help someone else, I help myself as well.

Reflection question:

- When is the last time you helped someone without any expectation of getting something back?
- How do you feel when your efforts to help someone go unnoticed or unappreciated? What does this reveal about your expectations in service?
- What motivates you to help others? Are you driven by a sense of duty, compassion, or something else?
- Have you seen suffering and tried to do something to improve the situation? Why or why not?
- In what ways do you practice detachment from the results of your actions? How does this influence your sense of fulfillment in helping others?
- What small acts of kindness or service do you offer in your daily life? How do these contribute to your understanding of Karma Yoga?

I encourage you to commit to taking at least one selfless action per week, to see where you can be of service and help.

These paths of yoga show us that in order to be truly well, we have to extend mutual respect and care to every being we are in relationship with. My sense is, if you become more mindful of the world around you and commit to reducing suffering for all, then it is yoga.

5

HOW THE TRAUMA OF COLONIALISM LIVES IN OUR BONES

UNDERSTANDING THE COLONIAL history of India is essential to understanding the way yoga is currently practiced in the West. In the dismantling cultural appropriation workshop I lead as part of a trauma-informed yoga teacher training, I always include information about India's colonial history.

A few days after leading this online training in 2022, I got an email from an Indian American student who had been in attendance. She wrote, "Sharing India's history of colonization was impactful. Most people don't give a damn about this important part of the history of yoga—in fact, most people don't care about *any* history of yoga unless they are forced to. Is this a part of the 200-hr Yoga Teacher Training? I know it was not when I did my training."

I could sense this student's anger. I have felt this same anger many times while researching and speaking on yoga's history. This expression of pain is a result of the colonial history of South Asia and the knowledge that yoga exists in a context of histories and legacies of colonialism. Our anger is valid. Our anger comes with a message.

How can anyone claim to love yoga as a practice and path so much and yet *know nothing about its history*?

When I go into different trainings and workshops, I try to start with an assumption of good faith, that yoga students and yoga practitioners mean well and are sincere. So perhaps it is not that they do not wish to know about the history but simply are ignorant and don't know about this history *yet*. While learning about yoga's colonialist history can bring about righteous anger for some, I've seen others react with resistance. This, too, is a way that colonialism still shows up in yoga spaces.

In that same workshop on dismantling cultural appropriation I mentioned earlier, I gave a list of ways students could work to acknowledge, understand, and see the ways they play into culturally appropriating yoga and how they might honor the roots of yoga. At the end, I asked everyone about one thing they were going change. One older white student raised her hand and said, "I always leave yoga classes before Savasana ends and after taking this workshop, I am going to stay through Savasana."

This felt like a shallow response to me. I wondered if she learned anything at all during the workshop. Yes, Savasana can offer a space for contemplation, reflection, rest, and integration, and it is vastly important. But this felt to me like the student listened at only a surface level and will continue to do whatever she wants. She deliberately chose to ignore the core message.

As strange as her response to the ideas I was presenting might seem, I have found that people are looking for a simple checklist of dos and don'ts for how to practice yoga: No longer saying "namaste" at the end of class. Check. Removing all statues and idols of Hindu gods and goddesses from the space. Check. Hiring one South Asian yoga instructor. Check.

Following a checklist like this is a distraction. It doesn't get to the heart of the issues and doesn't create enough contemplative space to uncover the colonialist implications of a white yoga practitioner wearing a bindi, putting on a Ganesh T-shirt, or pointing their feet toward a picture of Durga Mata.

Distraction, or diversion, is another response to confronting the colonialist history of yoga. In the same workshop, as I was teaching examples of cultural appropriation in yoga (e.g., making a profit or turning yoga into a business without any credit or acknowledgment of the source culture) I used CorePower as an example. I was sharing how CorePower's website has these quotes:

> *Trevor [the founder of CorePower] practiced a variety of yoga disciplines at yoga studios across the country & found an opportunity to make yoga dynamic, challenging, and convenient.*
>
> *And it wasn't long before people were talking about this new yoga.*

This was a case of a huge chain of yoga studios that has turned yoga into a for-profit exercise without acknowledging yoga's history or where it comes from. A white woman responded, "Trevor is the founder, not the CEO."

I had been referring to Trevor as the CEO of CorePower, and not the founder. I saw her message, took a deep breath, and knew this was a learning moment for us all.

I replied, "What I want us to notice here is how we are not focusing on the core issue of extraction and commodification but instead are fixating on my perceived mistake on Trevor's title. We are not focusing on how CorePower is adding to cultural appropriation of yoga but instead wanting to make sure we get his title right. This is bypassing the heart of the issue that is being raised."

At the end of the presentation, I honestly and openly shared how that comment had bothered me. How something like that happens time and time again to people of color. How our real issues are not listened to or heard, and instead something minor is centered.

To this woman's credit, she did privately message me later. She wrote: "Thank you for your time and learning. It was really well presented and informative. I apologize for triggering you with my input and correction. It wasn't my intention, but I could see how it could look distracting from the observation (which is warranted) and shifting the power dynamic. I hope to learn more from you in the future!" I never heard from her again.

Understanding history provides a container for us to move forward with intention. Many present-day world problems are a result of the colonial legacy. To come back to the heart of yoga as it originated in the source culture and restore it as a practice of liberation for all, we must confront yoga's painful colonialist past.

An Era of Darkness: India's Colonization by the British

The entire history of India's colonization by the British is beyond the scope of a single chapter. It is such a momentous and destructive period of history that it altered the course of several nations and millions of people's lives—to this day, in fact. Entire books have been written about it. (For further reading, I recommend *An Era of Darkness: The British Empire in India* by Shashi Tharoor.) However, for the purposes of our discussion, it is important to understand some of the broad strokes of this era of racist colonization and subjugation.

India's economy was once one of the largest and most powerful in the world. By the mid-twentieth century, an estimated $45 trillion had been stolen from the country and an estimated 100 million people had died from several famines, epidemics, riots, and slaughters. How did India go from one of the richest countries in the world to one of the poorest? We can look at the East India Company and the British Raj for that.

In 1613, the first British (East India Company) factory was set up in Surat, a city in the present-day western Indian state of Gujarat. However, what made this company different from others is that it had a large army; by the early nineteenth century, it was 250,000 strong, larger than that of many nations, and while the officers were British, the vast majority of company soldiers were Indian.

By 1757, the Mughal dynasty was going into decline. Seeing an opportunity to establish political dominance, the East India Company waged war on the ruling Nawab Siraj-ud-Daula of Bengal and seized control of the entire state. Robert Clive, a company man, became the governor of the state. He drained its wealth by charging local people to live there and diverting all its money to the British. The company went on to seize other parts of the country, including Delhi, the capital of the Mughal dynasty. Over the next several decades, the company, backed by the British government, colonized most of India through political corruption and outright violence.

In 1858, the British government ended company rule in India, and the country was transferred from the East India Company to the British Empire. Queen Victoria was proclaimed empress of India, and the British Raj began, ruling over almost all of modern-day India, Pakistan, and Bangladesh.

To maintain colonial rule, the Raj used strategies like "divide and rule" to pit Indians against one another. They made the existing Hindu oppressive caste system more rigid and deepened communal divides between Hindus, Muslims, and Sikhs. They deliberately sowed seeds of division among the masses along racial and religious lines, partly in retaliation after Hindus and Muslims cooperated during the 1857 mutiny.

The Hindu–Muslim divide was amplified after the First War of Independence in 1857 as a result of British prejudices, which ultimately led to the division of East and West Pakistan from India, multiple conflicts, and ongoing sectarian tensions.

In 1905, England divided Bengal into Hindu and Muslim sections, with different rules for the British and the Indians. Power and privilege preserved for the white supremacy was an essential feature of British colonialism, as it was for European colonial systems throughout history. Steve Martinot writes the following:

> *Whites did not simply gain racial supremacy within a field in which a number of races already existed;* ***they invented race as a system*** *in which they were already supreme, a field of definition in which other races were already inferior. Though*

> *"racism" is alleged to exist between other races than the white, all racialization has occurred with respect to white supremacy itself, as the inventor and generator of the concept of race, and thus all racism makes essential reference to "white racism."*

The denigration of Indian culture and language was part of the agenda. In 1835, the English Education Act redirected funds toward restructuring educational institutions—with the explicit objective of making English the predominant language of instruction and communication—and leading to the attempted erasure of many South Asian languages.

Between 1770 and 1947, an estimated thirty-five million Indians died in eleven massive famines as a direct result of failed British policy. One of the most atrocious examples is the Bengal Famine in 1943, which endured for slightly over a year, claiming the lives of millions and triggering a severe economic collapse. Instead of being allocated to aid the suffering masses, funds were diverted toward financing weapons and military supplies, exacerbating the poverty crisis.

On April 13, 1919, a horrendous event known as the Jallianwala Bagh massacre or the Amritsar massacre unfolded. In Amritsar, Punjab, British India, a large and peaceful Sikh crowd gathered at the park Jallianwala Bagh to protest British oppression and the arrest of pro-independence activists Saifuddin Kitchlew and Satyapal. The protesters were surrounded by buildings on three sides, leaving only one exit. The British positioned troops to block the exit and fired on the crowd. Even as the protesters desperately tried to flee, the troops continued firing until their ammunition was depleted. Fifteen hundred people or more are thought to have been murdered.

Despite the magnitude of this tragedy, Britain has never formally apologized for the massacre—although in 2019, it expressed "deep regret" for the event.

I remember learning about this massacre as an eight-year-old. My family and I were at the San Jose gurdwara, and they were showing a short film that went over these horrific details. I remember being shocked and deeply sad. How could someone commit such an atrocious crime against peaceful protesters? And near a sacred religious site like the Golden Temple, the Sri Harmandir Sahib. My first time in India, as a nine-year-old, we visited the site. You could still see the bullet-ridden walls and a well that people jumped into to escape the gunfire. There was an eerie quiet in the air as other people around me took in the site. The pain of this event was one that I and many others could *feel.*

By the time of India's independence in 1947, Britain was bankrupt in the wake of World War II. With no resources to continue its control, Britain wanted out and assigned the task of dividing India and Pakistan to Sir Cyril Radcliffe, *a lawyer who had never even been to India before and knew nothing of its history, society, or traditions*. Radcliffe drew up his maps in thirty-six days, dividing provinces, districts, villages, and homes, and promptly rushed back to Britain, never to return to India. The British showed little concern for the lives that would be lost as they quickly left.

But no one would tell Indians where those lines were drawn until the actual day of independence. This led to mass panic and chaos. An estimated fifteen million people were uprooted in one of the largest migrations in history, and between one and two million of them died because of large-scale communal violence, starvation, and disease. At least seventy-five thousand were raped and abducted. Muslims were forced to go toward East and West Pakistan, while Hindus and Sikhs went in the other direction. Families were split due to this forced migration, which was created by a British man who had never even visited India before drawing up his ill-considered map.

I've seen videos of elderly Sikhi men in turbans with long, white beards crying at the border between Punjab and Pakistan, finally reunited with their brother or sister or daughter after being forced to stay apart for fifty, sixty, or seventy years. It's heartbreaking to watch.

When I was nine years old, my dadaji told me that during the partition, he had to hide in a room in his house as police officers and others went around with guns, killing people. He heard the ringing of gunshots for hours.

This was only seventy-seven years ago. Living generations can remember it. This violence and trauma of forced migration is still carried in my body and in my genes. The same is true for all descendants, whether they are conscious of this inherited trauma or not. This violence is passed down and has changed DNA. The stains of this violence remain evident in modern-day South Asia and in current structures and systems of oppression and division.

The Impact of Colonialism on Yoga

The violence of colonialism had a direct impact on the practice of yoga. The British thought Hatha Yoga to be primitive, and people were forced to practice in secret. In some places, yoga was banned completely. People's ancestral and spiritual practices were taken away from them.

In her study of the history of yoga, Amara Miller states:

> *When British rule in India began in 1773, hatha yogis were actually viewed negatively by both Westerners and Indians. Hatha yogis were associated with black magic, perverse sexuality (based in tantric philosophy), abject poverty, eccentric austerities, and disreputable, sometimes-violent behavior. This wasn't simply prejudice, either. From the fifteenth century until the nineteenth century, highly organized bands of militarized yogis roamed Northern India, controlling trade routes and becoming so powerful that they were able to challenge the East India Company and British rule.*

There was a late eighteenth-century ban on armed militant ascetics—yogis who were warriors in North India. There were several different groups of ascetic warriors at that time, who occasionally fought with each other or were employed as mercenaries for hire. At times, they also resisted the British and maintained their own military and economic autonomy. The British banned them from being armed in order to consolidate their rule.

The British government also banned wandering yogis and tried to promote more "acceptable" religious practices among Indians—namely, the meditative Hinduism common among the educated, upper castes, and upper classes. These policies were supported by wealthier Indians who hoped for reconciliation with British rule and found traditional Hatha yogis disturbing at best. As the scope of colonial police powers grew in India, poor Hatha yogis were increasingly demilitarized and forced to settle in urban areas, where they often resorted to postural yogic showmanship and spectacle to earn money. As a result, physical Hatha Yoga practices became associated with the homeless and poor and were considered by both the British and Indians as "not only inferior but parasitic on other, worthier expressions of yoga that foregrounded meditative traditions."

Certain practices of yoga were socially accepted by the British, while other practices and lineages of yoga were ridiculed and oppressed. Colonialism and imperialism overwrite the stories of others, creating an oppressive environment, erasing people's histories, worldviews, and ways of being to the point that people internalize the narrative of the oppressor and unwittingly become agents of this pernicious agenda of erasure.

In my interview with Dr. Shyam Ranganathan, a researcher, scholar, author, and teacher of philosophy and an expert in the neglected traditions of Indian moral philosophy, we spoke about the impact of British colonialism on South Asia and yoga.

Dr. Ranganathan noted that in precolonial South Asia, people were free to adopt the philosophical views they wanted to. Disagreement was expected and common. Colonization is rooted in ancient Greek thought that "treats the tradition of white people as the judge or explanation of everything." South Asian spiritual practices were seen as a deviation from "normal" secular life.

"And so, people start creating all these stories about their religious identities," Dr. Ranganathan states, "which would simply not have occurred had there been no Western colonization. They would have just been talking about dharma and disagreeing about it without creating such strong separate identities." In other words, the colonial privileging of one religious perspective over another helped create conflict based on religion: Hinduism versus Buddhism versus Sikhism versus Islam, and so on.

Before colonization, there was much more overlap between what we refer to now as practicing Hindus, Muslims, Jains, Buddhists, and Sikhs. You could say there were Hindu Muslims, Sikhi Hindus, Buddhist Jains, et cetera. Yoga has always been tied to these theologies in some sense through the common understanding of karma, moksha, samsara, esoteric doctrines, scriptural texts, and so on. We can certainly say yoga is a part of pan-South Asian religious traditions—Hinduism, Buddhism, Jainism, and Sikhism—what we refer to now as dharmic religions. Yoga belongs to no particular religion.

Around the cusp of the fifteenth and sixteenth centuries, yoga was a thriving practice in pre-colonized India. It was an ideology that many practiced. The idea of religion is a Western (Eurocentric) creation.

Dr. Ranganathan puts it like this:

> *In other words, for the purposes of colonization, the British decided to rebrand a vibrant tradition of secular philosophical freedom into a religion, which would then have no part to play in the secular administration of South Asia. This move cements the subservience of the Indigenous philosophical tradition in South Asia to Western rule and conveniently exempts Western rule from non-Western moral criticism. The political purpose of creating "Hinduism" as a religion was to get rid of South Asian moral philosophy.*

Going Beyond Gender

Religion mixed with colonialism and patriarchy has oftentimes upheld misogyny and brought with it strict gender norms and ways that people had to conform. Powerful women and members of the LGBTQIA+ community have played major roles in yoga and in all faith traditions. However, many of their stories have not been recorded or have been intentionally erased. There have been yoginis and dakinis in both tantric and Buddhist yoga lineages who have heralded the way for their followers. Third gender people have often been revered throughout South Asian history, going back thousands of years before Muslim invasion, and are found in Hindu holy texts like the Ramayana and the Mahabharata, where Hindu hero Arjuna becomes the third gender. The most common are the hijras, who are generally referred to as the third sex, Tritiya Prakriti, which is neither male or female. Hijras are sometimes compared to sadhus, who also renounce their biological family, social/caste status, and sexual life to live with a guru and learn as a chela, or disciple, the ways of being. This is similar to any spiritual and yogic community in India where there is the guru–student lineage. This includes learning how to play ritual roles in blessing births, marriages, and more. As author Kristofer Rhude writes, "To many Hindus, it is the third gender nature of hijras—including their sacrifice of their procreative ability to the goddess—that grants hijras this incredible religious power." They are seen as having a special link between the human condition and God.

However, when the British colonized South Asia, they brought with them puritanical concepts and grossly limited ideas of gender, and they were shocked by the third gender people. The British named all hijras criminals in 1871. Hijras were marginalized and stigmatized. This law was repealed shortly after independence in 1947, but their place in society is still marked by discrimination. When my brother got married in India, and on another occasion when my cousin was having a baby, hijras came to our house in the village and gave their blessing through dance and song. I could acutely see how my family revered them and acknowledged the spiritual powers and connection that they hold. It is no different than turning to spiritual gurus for their blessing. This is a reminder that patriarchy and colonizers in historical times might try to say only men can be holders of faith or spiritual leaders, but this is incorrect.

Colonialism in the Past and Present

The twisted logic of colonialism is alive and well today. These systems of oppression work by making us believe we do not have a choice. That we are fated to feel less than and bound to our conditioning. These same systems purposely work to keep marginalized groups of people from growing, healing, and reaching their fullest potential.

These systems are diligently at work in the US Supreme Court and Republican Party to make abortion access illegal. They can be seen every time police officers brutally apprehend, assault, and murder those in brown and Black bodies. Their impact is evident in the way Indigenous peoples are denied governance and are forced to fight to rebuild a connection with their lands. This is the reality for too many people who live with ongoing legacy of colonialism—it forefronts race in the public perception about who is more worthy of our awareness, care, and support.

America has an ugly colonial history. Most of us who are not indigenous to these lands that make up North America—for instance, those of us living on Turtle Island, where I write these words or are the descendants of enslaved peoples—are uninvited settlers. We are living where Indigenous tribes were brutally murdered and their lands stolen by the British, French, Dutch, and Spanish, among other imperial forces. For those of us whose ancestors came to this land by choice from other places, it is important to acknowledge this history. This is settler colonialism.

Acknowledging the legacy of these harms requires us to have a safe container to hold our own fragility, vulnerability, resistance, denial, and wounds. We need the right emotional and contemplative space for our growth. This is challenging to uncover, learn, hold, and transform.

We cannot spiritually bypass these histories of colonialism and violence. We cannot "love and light" our way to understanding and resolution without seeing and understanding these histories clearly. Otherwise, they repeat themselves, causing great harm.

Yoga offers us contemplative practices to do this work, to touch the sadness and grief within. As one of my Buddhist teachers said, "We are all a little sad all the time and that's okay." And how could we not be? With all these histories of violence within us and the knowledge of our mortality?

This is encouragement to expand and grow your perspective to relate at a physical and emotional level to the reality of the suffering that prevails. When we take time to really feel that, it can help us to consider ways in which we might give back a little more, pray for our collective, or give our time and attention.

This is a choice we can all make: to not turn away from suffering by relating to ourselves and others in a way that might prompt a helpful response. Which parts of yourself are calling for your attention, for our loving awareness? Can you consider how other people you know or are aware of might need the same?

Being Suffocated by Colonialism: A Personal Story

As I started working on this chapter, I found myself completely stuck. For over two weeks, I could not get myself to sit down and write about colonialism. My anxiety escalated; my inner critic chastised me for stumbling. I really wanted to write, but something greater than me was causing so much resistance. In talking with my partner, friends, and therapist, I kept intellectualizing and pondering, *What is wrong with me?*

This growing anxiety bled into other areas of my life, which finally brought me to schedule a breathwork session with a facilitator I had worked with before. Fifteen minutes before the session, I took some time to write down my intentions for the session. I wanted to uncover what this crushing resistance was about. Why could I not write about this?

I hopped on Zoom, and we began with a body scan meditation. Once we moved into observing the chest and throat, I could feel a sense of *suffocation*, like I couldn't take a full breath, like I was drowning. It felt as though there was a dense weight on my lungs, restricting my capacity to breathe, to access my life force, to use my voice. My body was telling me that I *was not safe to share my story*. I felt tears rush to my eyes. Finally, I had clarity on why I had felt so stuck.

This is the impact of colonialism; it has a constricting force. I was struggling with the internalized idea that as a brown woman, I have to validate my humanity.

For centuries, colonized people and their descendants have not been able to breathe, have not been given their autonomy, and have had their power and lives taken away. Social, cultural, and political systems have made it so. As I write this, thousands of Palestinian people are being bombed and killed in a genocide in Gaza by the Israeli state while the mainstream media refuses to tell the full story, forcing those who are suffering to expose their pain in a desperate bid to be seen and heard.

Michelle C. Johnson, author of *Skill in Action*, says: "It is a radical act to breathe because oppression takes the breath away." Oppression crushes one's spirit and heart and makes people disconnected from their body, leaving in its wake depression, anxiety, fear, and post-traumatic stress disorder (PTSD).

I felt that crushing weight while writing this chapter, while writing this *book*. I felt that I needed a historian or academic to validate what I was saying. I thought that only then would I be taken seriously, as colonialism and patriarchy say that my lived experience is not enough.

That healing session made me realize that the constriction in my throat and chest was a visceral reaction to feeling the heaviness of this legacy. When I connected to that, I realized my connection to the people, including my own ancestors, who have been forced to give up their culture, their lands, their home, and have been subjected to unfathomable amounts of violence.

I was able to feel into the worth of my story and my role in speaking up for the millions of people who have had their breath and ultimately their lives taken away, through violence, genocide, murder, exploitation, and oppression.

Connecting Back to Our Bodies as Sacred

We've been socialized to live more in our minds than our bodies, to give more importance to intellect and logic. Many of us are taught to discount our feelings as silly, to see our intuition as "woo-woo," and to ignore our bodies even when they are begging for us to slow down, to check in and listen. I let my shoulders shake and my tears penetrate the depth of my sorrow for those of us still grappling with the effects of colonialism on our lives in the present day.

Oppression thrives off our disconnection. It teaches us a lie—that our bodies are only valuable *if an external body of authority deems them to be so*. The truth, however, is that we are already enough and our voices matter. There is medicine in each one of us that has the potential to heal one another and these lands.

I lovingly invite you to practice checking in with your body now.

You can experiment with placing one hand on your chest and one hand on your belly.

If it feels safe to do so, close your eyes or soften your gaze.

Roll your shoulders up to your ears and drop them back and down. Do this two to three more times, inhaling the shoulders up and exhaling them back and down.

It might feel nice to breathe in fully through the nose and sigh out through the mouth. Repeat if it feels good.

It is safe to breathe, to be here, to let go. Slowly invite your breathing into a natural rhythm and pace. Notice how your breath just is, how the body breathes, nourishing you with life—there is nothing you have to do.

Bring the awareness of your mind to any part of your body you might intuitively want to connect with. Perhaps it's your chest or your heart?

As you breathe into this part of your body, what does it have to say to you? Do you notice any sensations here? Is there a texture or color that arises? *Trust whatever comes up.*

Invite your body to speak to you. The message might come through as a thought, as a felt sense, as a somatic release through tears or shaking, as a visualization, as something you hear. Whatever comes up, give it space to do so.

Stay with this part of the body for as long as you wish. You may wish to move onto other parts of your body. Once you feel the practice is complete, I invite you to wrap your arms around yourself, and thank yourself, thank your body. You hold so much medicine within yourself, my love.

This is an exercise you may wish to revisit daily. During different periods of my life, it has been one I have turned to several times a day. It is profound to know, witness, and experience how much wisdom we embody.

6

UNPACKING OUR ROLE IN THE DECOLONIZATION JOURNEY

WHEN TALKING ABOUT the colonization and decolonization of yoga, we cannot focus on only Europeans and white supremacy. We must also look at India's legacies of harm, including caste, class, and religious hierarchies like Hindu supremacy and Islamophobia.

As a South Asian yoga practitioner and teacher in the beginning of my decolonizing yoga journey in 2019, I had a simplistic idea of what it meant to decolonize yoga. I was personally unraveling the layers through which I had internalized white supremacy and coming to terms with how much colonialism had messed up the world, which is a mammoth task in itself. I was looking at how the British had colonized present-day India and Pakistan, the enduring trauma, and then what it means to live as a Punjabi Sikh woman with brown skin, as an uninvited settler on Turtle Island, colonized as the United States. I was exploring how South Asians are erased in modern-day yoga, especially in the West.

One temptation of this discourse is binary thinking, which continues the dehumanizing narrative that separates us from them, the colonizer and colonized, the oppressor and the oppressed. When we dehumanize one another, we are not acting from a liberated space. This prevents the dialogue from moving forward.

The fact is that we *all* hold identities of oppressor and oppressed. India was colonized by the British and faced grave injustices and oppression—at the same time, within India, the caste system was (and is) alive. Brahmins, self-appointed to be at the top of the caste system, have throughout history used ideology to subjugate certain groups of people. This is the same for other upper caste people who followed the ideas of caste to marginalize those "underneath them."

The complicated truth is that we are all complicit in harm. We are either taking steps to dismantle the colonizer worldview that underpins society or we are a part of the problem.

As humans, we have to acknowledge that we are all liable to make mistakes. This admission creates spaces for natural human error to occur and for one to take accountability and repair harm. Mojdeh Cox speaks to what she calls *radical accountability*, which she defines as "getting to the fundamental root of one's responsibility" and "committing to the self-exploration required to understand how you may be contributing to the problem as an individual." Radical accountability is a compassionate approach toward self and others, building an ability to care for all people with the same level of empathy that we show to our most loved.

We need to find a way to invite in transformational healing justice. Otherwise, we recreate cycles of harm where people are not given a second chance to redeem themselves. All people, regardless of race, ethnicity, gender, or background, are equally capable of perpetuating injustice and contributing to cycles of harm. Within the context of yoga, South Asians have a responsibility to untangle the layers of violence caused through casteism, Hindu supremacy, Brahmanical patriarchy, and Islamophobia.

The Caste System in India

The caste (*varna* in Sanskrit) system has existed for a long time in many South Asian nations. It was created and put into place during the Vedic period, and over history it became more rigid and institutionalized. There are even mentions of the caste system in the Vedas and the Upanishads, where these texts laid out who was at the top and who was at the bottom. In the Vedas, four castes are outlined: the Brahmins (the priests/academics), the Kshatriya (the warriors/rulers), the Vaisya (the artisans/merchants/farmers), and the Shudras (the laboring class).

The fifth class is those with no caste identity such as the Dalits and tribal people. Beyond these, there were thousands of other castes. This caste hierarchy was sustained by texts that Brahmins wrote themselves. Dalits were treated horribly and not given the same rights or dignities as other people in the caste system—this continues in our present day. I recommend reading *The Trauma of Caste: A Dalit Feminist Meditation on Survivorship, Healing, and Abolition* by Thenmozhi Soundararajan and *Caste: The Origins of Our Discontents* by Isabel Wilkerson to learn more. Caste was made into a social, legal, and cultural law. Indignity and violence were made acceptable at a societal level. This is what happens when a group of people are first characterized and grouped together as an "other," which then permits further dehumanization.

When I visited my grandparents in Punjab as a child, we would have different people who cleaned the house, cooked, or did the laundry. I noticed that oftentimes, their clothing looked much simpler than what my family and I wore. When I asked my mom about it, she simply said they were of a different, lower caste than us and that was the job they were able to do. I remember wondering why we had so much support around us, and I felt uncomfortable that it felt so unequal. Growing up, I have also seen the prideful way that my family and others proclaim that they are Jatt. It was instilled in me that our status was something to celebrate and to be proud about, and this narrative is reinforced in Punjabi and Bollywood songs and movies.

I remember pointing out a mosque in my dad's pind (village) in Punjab a few years ago. My cousins explained that more Muslims were moving to Punjab and buying land. This was said in a neutral way, but I could tell my extended family had mixed views about this. That same year, Muslims were being targeted by the Bharatiya Janata Party (BJP), led by Narendra Modi, the prime minister of India, who has a Hindu nationalist stance. Seated in the courtyard of my dad's family home in Punjab, my uncle remarked, "Good! They should be taken out."

My mouth fell wide open. Before I had a chance to say something, my dad stepped in. He shook his head and replied calmly, "You can't think like that. Muslims are people exactly like us. And our gurus [of Sikhism] learned from Muslims and revered them too. Our gurus spoke about equality for all beings. We cannot celebrate the violence of other people because they have another faith. This goes against Sikhi tenets that accept all people regardless of their religion, caste, and creed."

I was surprised by the speed of my dad's response and agreed completely. To have such learned hatred to support the murder of Muslims was painful to see up close. My uncle looked uncomfortable and had nothing to say in return. Caste may have been removed from the laws, but it still exists in the cultural fabric of South Asia. Even though Sikhism was literally created to be anti-caste, caste is still *culturally* practiced and followed.

Brahmanical Appropriation

Some historians have pointed out that yoga was once appropriated by the Brahmin caste. Brahmins claimed yoga practices and texts as their own, and with the caste system positioned themselves as the top. Yoga wasn't allowed to be studied and practiced by all because not everyone could learn Sanskrit. Brahmins, being the highest caste, were the only ones allowed to learn and study Sanskrit and thus practice yoga—and only Brahmin men at that. Patriarchy rearing its head once again.

This appropriation cut against a diverse history of yoga practice and knowledge. Sanskrit, for instance, is not actually the only language in which yogic texts were written or communicated orally. During Buddha's period, it was the language of Pali, and there was also yoga knowledge communicated and written down in Tamil and more.

The caste system was created and cemented by yogic ideologies like karma and dharma. Those in charge used karma to say that, because of past deeds, people were now born into a certain caste. They then used dharma to say that it was the birthright of people of lower castes to fulfill their duty.

This is comparable to white supremacy, where structures are created to say that one group (white people) or class of people is better than another one. I'm reminded of the adage that history repeats itself. Today, Modi has developed a campaign that says that yoga is Indian and Hindu, to show India as a pure democratic peaceful place. International Yoga Day is one such campaign created by Modi. But yoga does not belong to one nation or religion. It is, in a sense, co-opting yoga's vision (one of peace and civility) to masquerade or hide how violent and power hungry the BJP and Modi are. In the last six years, Sikhs and Muslims have been targeted and killed by the BJP. This party is using violence to build a supremacist ideology and supremist political system that declares Hindus are the best and everyone else is underneath them.

The True Historical Diversity of Yoga

How are we to disentangle these histories of oppression in yoga? We can start by recognizing the true historical diversity of yoga—that yoga cannot be owned by any one group seeking power. Yoga is an Indigenous tradition. It predates caste and religion. Yoga originated in what was known at the time as the Indus Valley, which is now present-day Afghanistan, northwestern India, and Pakistan.

Later on, yoga was shaped and impacted by the religions that sprang up in this area. The dharmic religions of Hinduism, Buddhism, Jainism, and Sikhism all have spiritual practices and paths, and they are all known as yoga. Yoga has always adapted, evolved, and assimilated over thousands of years. I think this is one reason finding an inherently "pure" or authentic yoga path would be a fool's errand. Yoga has so many ideologies and different paths springing from it: Shramana, Buddhist, Tantric, Vedic, Bhakti, and more.

Once, feeling quite confused and down, I remarked to my Indian yoga teacher in Mumbai, "I feel like I have learned and am teaching a hodgepodge of yoga! Am I teaching properly, and what is true?"

My teacher smiled and said, "We have all been teaching hodgepodge yoga since the beginning of time."

The reason I say that yoga originated in South Asia and not India is to not center the nation of India and to encompass and acknowledge the other areas where yoga was practiced and studied. The modern states of South Asia include Afghanistan, Bangladesh, Bhutan, India, Maldives, Nepal, Pakistan, and Sri Lanka. Different forms of yoga, influenced by different religious traditions, have been practiced in these lands over the millennia.

The Harrapan Society

One of the world's oldest civilizations arose in the Indus Valley, extending from modern-day northeast Afghanistan to Pakistan and northwest India. The people of this region lived and farmed there as early as 7000 BCE, making up the Indus Valley civilization, also known as the Harappan Civilization. Between 3000 and 1900 BCE, this civilization was thriving, with flourishing urban centers like Harappa and Mohenjo-daro and other cities like Ganweriwala, Lothal, and Dholavira. These ancient peoples built well-planned cities with sophisticated urban planning, water sanitation systems, trade routes, and civil engineering, as well as a writing system that remains indecipherable to this day. It is thought that the Harappan peoples worshipped a mother goddess deity who symbolized fertility and that they most likely had a matriarchal society. Genetic studies indicate that the people in this area were a mixture of First Indians who arrived around sixty-five thousand years ago (out of ancient Africa) and early Iranian farmers.

When considering the earliest origins of yoga, we turn to this civilization. Seals over four thousand years old have been found in the Indus Valley sites with figures seated in a clear yogic posture. The most famous figure—seen in the Pashupati, or Proto-Shiva, seal—is seated with arms extended and resting on the knees in a classical meditative posture. When people say that yoga is a five-thousand-year-old tradition, they are referring to this seal as evidence. However, scholars have disagreed on what the seal is depicting. Some argue this is evidence that yoga has been practiced on the Indian subcontinent for over four thousand years, while others speculate it is not clear enough to say.

Evidence shows Harappans participated in a vast maritime trade network extending from central Asia to the Middle East. This leads me to believe if yoga or something similar was being practiced, it could have been shared from Egypt and other parts of the world even then. At this time, the Egyptian and Mesopotamian civilizations were also in existence. Carvings showing people in asana poses with depictions of the crown chakra and cobras, said to represent the two main nadis, have been found in Egypt, and research suggests that the first Egyptians were black-skinned and came from the Sudan, Ethiopia, and southern Arabia, as well as Babylon. Black and brown people have been exploring some form of yoga or spiritual and physical practice for thousands of years.

The Vedic Period

Around the decline of the Indus Valley civilization in 1900 BCE, new migrants known as the Aryans arrived. Exact origins of these Aryans are still debated by scholars, and ongoing research is being done. It is believed that the Aryans were either "Indo-Iranians (Persians) who merged peacefully with the Indigenous people of India (the Adivasis), intermarried, and were assimilated into the culture" or Indo-European tribes with origins around the Black and Caspian Seas, in the Central Asian steppes of southern Ukraine, Russia, and Mongolia. The Aryans brought horses, animal sacrifices, and their reverence of the cow. Through assimilation, a new Indo-Aryan culture emerged in this region. This marks the beginning of the Vedic period, from 1500–500 BCE, and is the earliest era in South Asia with written records for how yoga evolved. It is important to note that Adivasis (the Indigenous people of India) and Dravidians were already in the Indus Valley before the Aryans' arrival.

During the Vedic period, the earliest scriptures that would come to form the foundation of Orthodox Hinduism, the Vedas, were composed: the *Rig Veda*, *Sama Veda*, *Yajur Veda*, and *Atharva Veda*. The Vedas are considered among the oldest, if not the oldest, religious scriptures in the world, composed between 1500 and 1000 BCE. The Vedas lay out hymns, prayers, and proper religious rituals as a way to connect to the divine and provide principles for social organization (the varna, or caste system).

Yoga as a word first appears in the *Rig Veda*, although with reference to the "yoking" of the horses to the chariot of war. In this instance, we see yoga defined as "to yoke," not necessarily as a spiritual tradition. However, the *Rig Veda*—namely, the Kesin Hymn 10.136—suggests there were yogi-like ascetics on the margins of the Vedic landscape. The Kesin are described as wandering folk in tattered orange robes who are equally at home in the physical and spiritual worlds.

The Upanishads, also known as the end of the Vedas, mark the shift from external ritualistic focus of the early Vedic texts to an internal, contemplative exploration of spiritual truths. During the early Vedic period, we see rituals in which animals and other items are offered into fire to various gods for the purposes of obtaining worldly boons—special power, offspring, victory over enemies, et cetera. This is where the use of ahimsa first comes in, as a way to offer nonviolence to animals, to stop sacrificing them. The Upanishads provide profound insights into the nature of existence, consciousness, and the path of spiritual realization. These texts are concerned with understanding the nature of ultimate reality, known as Brahman, through the cultivation of knowledge for self-realization (atma jnana); these techniques are called yoga. The Maitri Upanishad, dated to around 500 BCE, includes specific limbs of yoga, such as pranayama, dhyana, dharana, tarka (inquiry), and samadhi.

The Sramanic Tradition

Corresponding to this period (around 500 BCE), we have the rise of renunciant ascetics, known as the Sramanic traditions (strivers), who developed independently to Brahmanical Vedic traditions. These included Buddhists, Jains, and Ajivikas. They were concerned with finding ways to bring an end to the cycle of rebirth (samsara) and the karma-driven suffering that characterizes human existence, and they developed techniques of meditation (dhyana) to lead to the ultimate goal of nirvana or moksha. These ideas that make up the spiritual core of yogic teachings made their first appearance in Sramanic traditions and were later incorporated into Vedic teachings. According to some scholars, the indigenous practices of the Indian subcontinent are preserved through Sramanic traditions, which they suggest may even precede Vedic traditions. Ascetics in the Sramanic traditions engaged in practices known as tapas to still the mind and burn away past karma—this can be seen in pictures of yogis holding one or both of their arms up for years. This is seen in comparison to the early Vedic ascetics, who practiced tapas to win boons of superpowers and material successes.

Over time, we see many different schools and ideologies of yoga, whether Vedantic, Puranic, Vaisnava, Saivite, Sramanic, Buddhist, or Tantric. They are different approaches to salvation. Later, we have introductions to texts like the epic Mahabharata, the Yogacara Buddhism textual corpus, and Patanjali's Yoga Sutras (in that order). Patanjali is one of the first to systemize different schools of yoga and put them into one text—he is not the inventor or founder of yoga, simply the compiler. While the Yoga Sutras were developed as a Brahmanical text for celibate Brahmin men at the time, Patanjali systemized preexisting traditions that pulled from Sankhyan philosophy, Yogacara Buddhism, the Mahabharata, Sramanic traditions, and more. There has never been one uniform school of yoga: "There was a plurality of variants and certainly different conceptualizations of meditative practices that were termed *yoga*."

Yoga, at this time, was a cluster of techniques that overlapped and merged with various traditions such as the knowledge-based traditions we looked at earlier, providing these philosophical systems with a practical method for attaining an experience-based transformation of consciousness.

From 600 to 1300 CE, yoga was important in a range of traditions—Saiva, Vaisnava, and Buddhist (that would later form Vajrayana Buddhism)—which were considered the dominant "religion" during this time and which we can understand as tantra. Tantra yoga is one of the first times we encounter chakras (wheel-like patterns of energy), the subtle body of prana and nadis, kundalini, and the systematic movement of energy through the channels. We see practices of subtle body cultivation and bodily alchemy. The idea of a network of subtle energy channels (nadis) is found as far back as the Brhadaranyaka Upanishad; however, it increases in sophistication and complexity in the tantric tradition, in the 500 CE text Nisvasatattvasamhita and then the 100 CE text Kubjikamatatantra, which lays out the six energy centers (the chakras). This period is important because we see the physical and subtle body begin to take more importance.

The Bhakti movement arose during this time to challenge the caste hierarchy established by Brahmins and to emphasize individuals' ability to connect to the divine directly. The Brahmin supremacy was challenged by saint poets such as Kabir, Ravidas, and Nanak.

Dharmic Religions

It is also important here to orient yoga in its geographical and cultural location. Four main religions originated in South Asia—Hinduism, Buddhism, Jainism, and Sikhism, along with hundreds of denominations. In this context, we can understand religions as spiritual traditions, and the spiritual path of all these dharmic religions can be called *yoga*. Each religion or spiritual tradition has its own holy books, saints (yogis), ideas of "God," "yoga," philosophies, rituals, traditions, symbols, et cetera.

As Prasad Rangnekar mentioned in his Finding Clarity workshops, the fundamental tenets and what these four religions have in common are as follows:

- There exists a limited mundane existence and a transcendental or sacred "truth."

- Yoga is the process to go beyond these limitations.
- Freedom is called *moksha/nirvana*, which is the end goal from samsara.
- Belief in the laws of karma and dharma is necessary.
- Yoga is not a path of self-serving spirituality—surrender, devotion, and love are important to go beyond oneself.
- A guru is essential and can be more of a principle than a specific person.
- Ethical and moral guidelines are a foundation.
- Realization is more important than theoretical knowledge.

This is important to understand when we think about where yoga originated and the common geographical roots and ideologies of the four main religions at the time in the Indian subcontinent. This path and the four religions speak of helping others and benefiting humanity.

During a mentorship session, Sri Prasad Rangnekar shared that all of the over ten thousand scriptures/books on yoga share the same thing: how to realize yourself. It is necessary for us to become our own autonomous beings. As Dr. Ranganathan shared in his book, *Yoga-Anticolonial Philosophy*, "Actual Yoga Practice is decolonial, as it is a practice of Devotion to Sovereignty that yields autonomy. One cannot be colonialized when one is autonomous, and colonialism aims to swap Isvara—everyone's Sovereignty—with the interpretation of a narrow worldview. Thus, the true practice of yoga serves as an act of resistance to colonization because it cultivates personal freedom and inner sovereignty, countering the oppressive forces of colonial rule."

Orienting Ourselves Toward Decolonizing Yoga

I have learned that the decolonial framework "does not mean a shift to pre-coloniality, for precolonial is not synonymous with anti-colonial." South Asians have also created and perpetuated their own systems of oppression before European colonization, via Brahmanical patriarchy, Hindu nationalism, and Islamophobia. So, what would we be returning to if we looked at decolonizing yoga as returning to the time before British colonization? Again, just layers of violence and oppression.

I turn to Philly-based activist and yoga and healing justice teacher Dr. Sheena Sood for a definition of *decolonization* here. Decolonization is a process of Indigenous cultures reclaiming self-determination and rights over their lands, governments, and regimes. I understand it to be a long-term process of Indigenous communities divesting and healing from the cultural, spiritual, linguistic, and psychological damage that endures due to colonial structures. I invite readers of this book to read Dr. Sood's two journal articles on this topic: "Towards a Critical Embodiment of Decolonizing Yoga" and "Cultivating a Yogic Theology of Collective Healing: A Yogini's Journey Disrupting White Supremacy, Hindu Fundamentalism, and Casteism."

While periods of coexistence existed between various Indian belief systems, these were not without conflict. However, the violence inflicted by European colonizers through their material and cultural domination far surpassed any internal disputes. Notably, the seemingly neutral term "Hindu" is itself a colonial construct by the British. It originated in the West and homogenized a multifaceted, multicultural civilization. Literally, *Hindu* simply refers to those residing east of the Indus River.

As we can see, yoga's lineage is interwoven with narratives of both the colonized and the colonizer. We are presented with a choice: to accept these inherited stories or to use them as a springboard for uncovering deeper truths. A commitment to dismantling ancestral histories of oppression necessitates a parallel commitment to revealing the multiplicity of these truths. By refusing to acknowledge the presence of violence and oppressive brutality within yoga's own history, we forfeit an opportunity, for ourselves and future generations, to transform into the most liberated versions of ourselves.

Liberating Yoga Framework

Here is a liberating yoga framework that I think would make a big impact if we practiced and taught in this way. The framework of liberation in yoga means using yoga to free ourselves from external sources of oppression as much as internalized oppression (e.g., tone policing ourselves). It means bringing light to these issues and then helping to free others.

This framework challenges the appropriation of yoga and the reduction of this ancient holistic system to a sport for the elite and wealthy, where it is misused as a pacifying tool to make people better producers in capitalism or as a feel-good modality as an individualistic pursuit.

A liberating yoga practice helps to build courage, confidence, and strength to do good in the world and to stand up to systems rooted in colonialism, capitalism, racism, and cisheteronormativity. A world built on the latter foundations, as we know, is scary, dangerous, and a depressing place to live. It's not an individual's fault that they can't make enough money to pay all their bills. Why do teachers in America get paid little while venture capital "bros" make millions? What does that say about what we value in our society? Kids are being shot at in schools. Racism is rampant. Anti-trans bills are being proposed and passed in the US government.

Our world is broken. Our society is broken. A liberatory yoga practice is one that considers the prevalence of this suffering.

Siddhartha Gautama the Buddha is one of my guides. He attained liberation at the age of thirty-five and then committed the rest of his forty-five years on this earth to helping others become free of suffering. Guru Nanak is my other model for liberation. He learned from many different teachers of Islam, Hinduism, yoga, Bhakti, and Sufism, after which he founded Sikhism with a view for equality for all. That is liberatory practice and revolutionary. Kali Ma is another one of my guides. I often reflect on her powerful image—her tongue thrust out, adorned with skulls, blood dripping from her form, her ten arms poised and fierce. She embodies intensity and strength, always ready to strike down evil and dismantle the forces of oppression. Kali, known as the "devourer of time," requires deep reverence because she is a radical goddess, one who will ruthlessly cut away all that is unnecessary. Invoking Kali means calling forth profound transformation, and one must understand how to honor and hold her energy with respect, as she reveals the raw truth and demands courage in the face of our own illusions. She is not someone to call upon carelessly.

A liberatory yoga practice:

- is one that acknowledges that Black and brown people have stewarded and been practicing yoga for thousands of years. We bow to these teachers, rishis, sages, saints, forest and cave dwellers, practitioners, enlightened ones, and yogis before us for their dedication, devotion, and teachings. For keeping these teachings alive through persecution, colonization, violence, in a simulation. Without them, we would not be able to walk on this path ourselves.
- is one that honors the land, the Indigenous stewards—past, present, and future—and seeks to protect and care for the land and work with Indigenous folks to give them back governance and stewardship over the land. It's recognizing that we are made up of the same elements that make up the land and work toward regeneration and combat exploitation of the land. It recognizes Indigenous and Native folks as the rightful owners and caretakers of these lands—of Turtle Island.
- is one that pays respect and builds a connection with our ancestors. For their struggles and gifts. Because without them, we would not be here. It seeks to know that we are not alone and we are supported by the loving embrace and courageous wisdom of our ancestors. It also works to acknowledge the harm that our ancestors may have caused and work to repair it, so that patterns of oppression and harm are not duplicated.

- is one that wishes to see all people free, regardless of race, gender, religion, caste, class, skin color, socioeconomic status, sexual orientation, disabilities, and physical and mental capability. It recognizes that there are real systems of oppression and inequalities that keep all people from being free, of accessing healthcare, education, fair compensation, and dignity. It recognizes that colonialism is the root of this oppression, inequality, and violence. It requires the practitioner to learn, unlearn, and be a part of systemic change.
- is one that can hold multiplicities of truth and work with *both/and*. It is a practice that honors the transformation/liberation potential of yoga *and* the oppression flowing through these histories and path. This requires a practitioner to be okay sitting with confusion, discomfort, existential angst, and disillusionment as truths are unraveled and growth is worked toward.
- is one that invites us to be gentle, compassionate, patient, and curious with ourselves. To know that this path of self-discovery will not always be easy and we must be kind to ourselves throughout the process. It is one that asks us to cultivate a kind inner voice because we have been taught by others to be hard on ourselves. This gentleness and tenderness is crucial in liberatory work. We do not wish to recreate inner systems of policing and hurting ourselves—instead love yourself as deeply as you can.
- is one that honors ancestral, cultural, and spiritual traditions, rituals and practices and knows that these hold deeply healing and powerful medicines. It recognizes that Black and brown people do not have to be validated, scientifically proven, clinically tested or whitewashed to be accepted as true and worthy of healing. It gives stewardship, credibility, and voice back to Black and brown people.

- is one that reminds us we are more than our bodies, minds, professional titles, possessions, and status in society. We are Divine beings having human experiences and deserving of dignity, care, love, and community. We know that there is more than we can see with our eyes and recognize the mystery that is spirit.
- is about liberating consciousness. If yoga is about being in a state of pure consciousness, then liberating yoga is about liberating consciousness from the confines and grips of hatred, fear, and apathy. From the confines and grips of capitalism, colonialism, patriarchy, and racism. Anything that keeps us separated and disconnected from ourselves, each other, and this planet.
- is one that endeavors to make all students feel included, accepted, seen, and heard. It sees yoga community as more than an hour-long fitness class. It builds solidarity and comradeship.
- is one where practitioners, students, and teachers work to make conditions better for all beings and especially for oppressed peoples. It recognizes our social and moral duty to care for one another. Where social justice, collective liberation, and social good is something we all strive for.

A liberatory yoga practice also understands that we need to be resourced. That's why we have our sadhana—a practice that anchors us into faith, purpose, and clarity. That's why we have sangha—people who care about us, can celebrate with us, and help us when we are beaten down and sad. Those that can mirror back to us when we might be heading down the wrong path. Those that will fight for and with us.

Solidarity and power in numbers is crucial. That's why we have these teachings—to keep us in integrity, in ethics, and in wisdom. To turn to teachers and texts that have been here before. To shed light when the path looks/seems dark and confusing.

I always end my classes with gratitude and merit, and I have shared my closing statement below.

In gratitude to the blessing of this life—the reality of all the highs and lows. In gratitude to the wisdom of these practices, in gratitude to the teachers and practitioners who have walked this path before us, illuminating it so we know that we are never alone. In gratitude to ourselves for making this very intentional time, space, energy, and commitment to practice. In gratitude for these lands for holding us.

May all beings everywhere with no limit be happy, healthy, safe, and at ease. May all beings be at peace and be free. (This is how we share the merits of our practice with all beings. This is the practice of metta from Buddhism.)

7

YOGA MATS, YOGA PANTS, AND EXPENSIVE CLASSES

DID YOU KNOW that you don't need a yoga mat to practice yoga? One of my yoga teachers, who has been practicing for over thirty-five years, told me he didn't even know what a yoga mat was until about ten years ago, when he showed up for a class and people were pulling them out. The truth is you could practice asana on any surface.

There's no need to have mats, blocks, straps, wheels—or yoga pants, the invention of which is one illustration of how capitalism has appropriated yoga. Companies came in and decided practitioners needed to dress a certain way to practice. Now we see yoga pants as leggings or tights that come in a wide assortment of colors and patterns. This idea of "yoga pants" was created by and first sold by Lululemon in 1998. Lululemon literally was founded to capitalize on yoga (asana) accessories. Nature provides us with what we require to survive, while society influences what we believe we desire.

One of my first yoga teachers in Delhi, an older woman who was also an Ayurvedic doctor, told us that we should wear loose-fitting clothing made out of cotton to practice asana, pranayama, and meditation because it breathes better and doesn't constrict the physical body. This is the opposite of what we see in most yoga studios and across mass media and social media.

Yoga has become a product in the capitalist economy. It is sold as a constant and relentless self-improvement project. To become the highest version of yourself, you have to be constantly taking yoga classes, signing up for courses, and of course, buying lots and lots of expensive products. As bell hooks shared in her book, *All About*

Love, "Keeping people in a constant state of lack, in perpetual desire, strengthens the marketplace economy."

Lululemon is a prime example of a company and brand swooping in to make billions of dollars from the commodification of yoga. Yoga is sold as an elite economic and social practice. Lululemon as a brand represents a certain level of status and elitism.

Lululemon has sold products like Mula Bandha thongs, a shirt with three white stripes on it representing Om Namah Shivaya (the words of a popular Hindu mantra), and $108 mala beads for meditation. This is cultural appropriation mixed with commodification and sheer audacity! The mala beads even had the Lululemon logo on them. I found a product review of the beads that said, "I love them. . . . They are beautiful and I feel very zen when I wear and use them. They calm me down and help me focus on the moment. A tad pricy but love, love them. Not sure why the other reviews are so negative. They must not be using their beads for the intended use. Peace and Love :)"

The line "They must not be using their beads for the intended use" is what really got me. As yoga practitioners, students, and teachers, people are still allowed to pass judgment and have discernment over what is happening in the world. Especially in relation to overpriced exoticized mala beads to adorn the costume or cosplay of a "Zen yoga teacher." Using these practices as a way to shut people up or to pacify them is antithetical to the original intentions and goals.

The Problems with the Commodification of Yoga

The problems with the commodification of yoga are many. For one, companies with lots of money, social sway, and advertising potential are able to create a false picture of what an "ideal" yoga practitioner ought to look like. This ideal is often presented as a thin young affluent able-bodied white cis woman. This isn't my ideal. When I think about a yoga practitioner, I think about someone who is much older than me, has life experience, is compassionate and socially minded, is comfortable in their body no matter its shape, and has kindness in their eyes. Someone who is comfortable with themselves and their personal weak spots—no one is perfect, and I appreciate authenticity and vulnerability. One of my teachers says the epitome of spiritual kindness for him is an old Indian woman with some teeth missing. This is not whom we see in Lululemon ads.

Another problem is that these companies are profiting from people's insecurity and search for well-being. Lululemon is one of many that charge hundreds of dollars for products and services that offer peace of mind. As yoga and mindfulness grow in popularity, so does the opportunity to capitalize on them. Companies and people plunder the "other" for cultural resources and then repackage and rebrand them for their own profit. *Eat Pray Love* comes to mind here, where other "faraway lands" and cultures get exoticized and construed for the white gaze. It also shows up as a white woman "falling in love" with chai while visiting India and then turning it into a profiteering enterprise.

Accumulating and flaunting wealth has nothing to do with being a yogi. In traditional yoga, you can have it or not have it—wealth, possessions, whatever. It does not matter. Your success as a yoga practitioner is not defined by how much you have accumulated materially or how "successful" you are.

Age-old wisdom reminds us that we are already whole and our highest self. This work of self-inquiry and reflection, practice, and application of the teachings highlights the ways we have lost sight of or abandoned the wholeness of our being. There is truly nothing that needs to be purchased to realize this. I wholeheartedly believe if we loved (and accepted) ourselves, overconsumption would be severely reduced.

I have seen how I have felt swayed to purchase cuter (more expensive) workout clothes to fit in with others at the yoga asana classes. To purchase a yoga mat from a certain brand because it is perceived to be better—to see it as an investment in becoming my best self.

To purchase a mala and singing bowl to play the part of an idealized yoga student and teacher.

Social media also creates this archetype of the ideal yoga practitioner as someone who can contort their body in different ways, someone who is always happy and peaceful, someone who lives a #blessed life. This can be very seductive for those looking for their place in the world. Projecting this image creates social capital and a convenient aspiration. However, this is just another illusion and a form of clinging, another pitfall of the commodification of yoga. As a yoga practitioner and teacher, I can say I still have all the same problems and struggles others have. Yoga doesn't get rid of those things because they are naturally occurring in life, and many problems are a result of systemic oppression. But yoga *does* provide tools to help move through these difficulties with more ease, mindfulness, and understanding. Those tools don't require fancy clothes or equipment. We can come to the understanding that suffering (dukkha) is a part of life and something we can hold with greater equanimity.

One way that I have personally moved away from playing into this social media idealization of the "perfect" yoga practitioner is reducing the number of posts where I am in asana shapes. I also share more about my story and my struggles so that people know that becoming a yoga practitioner, student, or teacher doesn't mean you automatically become a perfect human. If anything, yoga highlighted to me what a neurotic person I am and how often my perspective is incorrect!

In the traditional writings about yoga, Siddhis are defined as magical powers one can achieve through the practice of yoga. However, even here the teachings say to not get seduced by this achievement. We are warned not to practice yoga only to gain powers to make our faces more beautiful or attain more wealth. The purpose of yoga is not what we can *get*.

I am reminded of the yamas of Brahmacharya and Aparigraha. Brahmacharya teaches us to not overdo anything, such as the consumption of material things—a concept close to the idea of moderation.

Aparigraha, the teaching of non-greed and nonattachment, points to being content with what we have and not being envious of what others have or coveting those things. It means letting go of the attachment to wants and things. This also reminds me of the Buddhist teaching of the Middle Way. Yes, we can work to attain material items, *and* there can be a limit imposed as well. We are not calling for people to renounce everything and become cave dwellers or to demonize money. We must find a healthy balance of living in this world, where we need money to survive and thrive. Nonattachment is not necessarily about getting rid of your possessions. Rather, it's about not letting your possessions own you.

This also makes me think about fast fashion—particularly companies like Shein, where you can buy items for less than five dollars—and how these companies are a leading cause of creating unnecessary trash for the world. Do we really need to buy that eighth swimsuit? And I say this to myself as well! We are all interconnected to one another and to nature. Our choices and actions make an impact. This goes for luxury companies as well, who are not any more sustainable than fast fashion companies.

According to almost all schools of Indic thought, including Buddhism and Jainism, the more we desire, the more we are frustrated. The more we are frustrated, the more we strive to remove our frustration with sensory stimuli. And the more we strive, the more we damage ourselves and our environment and perpetuate our samsaric (unsatisfactory) existence. It is in the critique of this mindset of consumption that Patanjali claims to offer an alternative that remains perennially relevant to human existence.

We must learn to be satisfied with what we have instead of being stuck in a cycle of discontentment, which breeds desire.

One of my Buddhist teachers had us repeat over and over, "I am totally satisfied right now." I invite you now to repeat this to yourself, silently or aloud, at least ten times and really tune into the meaning behind what you are saying.

During a conversation with my friend Puja Singh—a queer artist, yoga teacher, and phenomenal kirtan singer—we reflected on how many courses and certifications we've taken to better ourselves. I've taken courses in trauma-informed yoga and Kundalini yoga; I've taken 200- and 300-hour yoga trainings. Puja, meanwhile, has become more advanced in kirtan. This is partly Svadyaya and provides an avenue to study, learn, and grow. I have seen how much I have changed from the beginning of a course to the end, and most times the transformation is positive.

However, this becomes tricky when we think the only way to spiritually advance is to continue taking course after course, reading book after book, and picking up certifications—in Reiki, sound bowl healing, womb healing, and the list goes on. Of course, each of these opportunities comes with a financial cost. Each is a product we purchase to improve ourselves. There needs to be ample time to digest, process, and integrate the teachings. Otherwise, we are left with borrowed wisdom. Borrowed wisdom is not the same as realized wisdom. The yogis knew this. That is why yoga is an experiential path.

Puja said, "Someone's spiritual practice and training could be to contemplate and meditate on 'Who Am I?' every single day, and that would be enough."

America's Obsession with Advertisements

When I lived in Brisbane, Australia, for two years, I was surprised and pleased to see the relative absence of advertising. I wasn't subject to billboards with ads on each corner, television programming didn't seem to have quite as many commercials, and stores closed earlier than they do in the US. Brisbane is where I worked through my personal shopping addiction and learned to spend more time in nature.

Living in America, I find advertising and consumerism to be a larger part of everyday life, even intruding into spaces I consider sacred. I was aghast a few weeks ago when I was hanging out at Santa

Monica Beach after a yoga workshop, and a small plane with a banner advertisement for Bud Light flew by. Shortly after, another plane with a banner for something else followed. Exasperated, I turned to my friends and said, "I can't even enjoy the blue skies without an advertisement! Is no real estate sacred? Is everything up to be commodified and subverted by capitalism?" The short answer, here, is *yes*.

Here's another practice: Begin to notice how many advertisements you come across in a day. And how many of them you did not give your explicit permission to view and consume. These ads subconsciously make us want to consume and desire things. Our awareness and attention and desire are a currency up for auction.

Economic agendas and ideologies are shaping our spiritual worldviews. Capitalism is pervading our lives and our thinking. We are products of capitalism. I sincerely hope we can undo that to some degree, and I think the first step is to at least become aware of it. Yoga can be a step toward that awareness.

New Age Spirituality

In America, spiritual enlightenment has been tied up with success, beauty, fitness, and wealth since the early nineteenth century. And the appropriation of yoga and South Asian thought and spirituality is a part of this history.

Take, for example, the transcendentalist movement, led in part by writers Ralph Waldo Emerson and Henry David Thoreau. Both shared a love for the ideas in works like the Bhagavad Gita and used Indian mythologies in their thinking.

Or take the story of William Atkinson, attorney, author, occultist, and pioneer of the American New Thought movement. Atkinson spoke of things like will manifestation, the law of attraction, the power of positive thinking, and the divinity of health, power, wealth, and success. As scholar and filmmaker Vivek Bald states in his article "American Orientalism," Atkinson wrote an estimated one hundred books, many of them under the Indian and Hindu pseudonyms of Yogi Ramacharaka, Swami Bhakta Vishita, and Swami Panchadasi. All his books on yoga are still in print today. In his books, he mashes up oriental occultism, divination, and mediumship—not speaking to what Hinduism or yoga really teach and believe. The New Thought movement promoted the belief that we can use our mind and positive thinking to change ourselves and the world around us—that you are able to get what you want if you are able to control your mind; right thinking has a healing effect.

The New Thought movement accumulated wisdom and philosophy from a variety of origins, such as ancient Greek, Roman, Egyptian, Chinese, Taoist, Vedic, Hindu, and Buddhist cultures and their related belief systems, primarily regarding the interaction between thought, belief, and consciousness in the human mind, and the effects of these within and beyond the human mind. There is a mish-mashing that happens here, all tied up with American capitalism. *Well-being through accumulating wealth.*

These famous New Age spiritual teachers glorify wealth, privilege, power, and individualism while ignoring systems of oppression. As bell hooks explains in her book *All About Love*, "Consider New Age logic, which suggests that the poor have chosen to be poor, have chosen their suffering. Such thinking removes from all of us who are privileged the burden of accountability. Rather than calling us to embrace love and greater community, it actually requires an investment in the logic of alienation and estrangement."

To me, this is the workings of capitalism and individualism, intersected with New Age thought and spirituality. This type of thinking says that because I have worked hard and manifested correctly using my mind, I have through *my own sheer will* created *my* fortune and success. Those poor people have chosen to be poor through their lack of discipline, hard work, and incorrect thinking.

This completely ignores histories of exploitation. How did your ancestors come to acquire their wealth? Was it through the forced labor of Black and brown people? Or lands stolen through the murder of Indigenous peoples? This New Age thought ignores how privilege and power lead to nepotism. It ignores how history and systems of oppression have created traps of inequality. This type of thinking removes the burden of accountability—that we need to listen to one another and share with those around us to reduce the rising inequalities. It makes me think of a story a dear friend shared with me about how Thich Nhat Hanh, a Vietnamese Thien Buddhist monk and peace activist, spent two days with a wealthy person who kept bragging about all he had. Finally on the second day, Thich turned to this gentleman and said kindly, "You think *you* made this all happen, huh."

The New Age movement in the US and UK really took off in the 1960s and 1970s, made up of white people from middle- and upper-middle-class backgrounds reacting to 1950s socioreligious conservatism. You can think of the "spiritual but not religious" folks here. New Age spirituality is often a combination of Black, Indigenous, and people of color (BIPOC) wisdom, traditions, and religions that have been blended into universal teachings where the goal is self-actualization and spiritual authority of the self—basically, it begins and ends with the individual. New Age spirituality has liberally taken and profited from Asian, Indigenous, African, African American, and South American cultures. This leads to loss of lineage, centering of the white colonizer worldview and the appropriation of these practices for an agenda that is antithetical to spirituality in its truest sense.

Dampening Our Attachment to the Consumer Mentality

Yoga is a path that helps us to abandon the consumer mentality. This can be done through the practice of all eight limbs of yoga, laid out by Patanjali in the Yoga Sutras, beginning with the yamas and niyamas to map out an ethical and moral framework.

I turn to Pratyahara here, the fifth limb on Patanjali's eight-fold path, which is often understood as the withdrawal of senses to go inward. I encourage all practitioners to learn to detach from the constant bombardment of sensory information and external distractions, such as external messaging and advertisements. By turning the senses inward, you are able to understand your own needs and thoughts better. The consumer mentality wants us to be externally tuned in so we continue seeing, and desiring what we see.

A practice I offer here is to set your phone's timer for five to ten minutes. Close your eyes or soften your gaze while looking at something a few feet away and begin to focus on your breath. Bring your attention to the natural in and out of the breath. Nothing to do here but observe your breath as a lifelong friend and companion, using the breath as an anchor for the mind, to shift the awareness from external stimuli to the internal world. Stay here for as long as you are comfortable and able, possibly until your timer goes off. This is a way to practice Pratyahara, to shift from being constantly externally facing to internally tuned in.

Our eyes are constantly seeking, searching, and comparing. And the way that yoga is marketed plays into that—becoming part of the problem rather than the solution. We see a certain ideal curated for us, a way to be a "perfect" practitioner, student, or teacher. I want us to dismantle this image, to know that the only "things" needed to be on this path are dedication, sincerity, and humility.

Yoga Sutra 2.7 reads, "*sukhānuśayī rāgaḥ*," which translates to "Attachment stems from [experiences] of happiness." This sutra speaks to the third klesha of raga, or of attachment. How we attain happiness from things and then how we begin to form an attachment to things (really anything here) that we believe bring us happiness. We get attached to anything that brings us pleasure because we want to keep feeling that way. We keep running after impermanent things for happiness.

So, what is a yoga practitioner, student, and teacher to do? I turn to Asteya here, the niyama that teaches us to not steal and to be mindful of not taking more than you need or are offered. We can become more aware of our choices in what we consume, want, need, and desire. Some questions to explore here:

- What are you desiring right now? Where does this desire originate from?
- How does your consumption impact yourself, others, and the planet?
- Do you believe a fruitful yoga practice is contingent on having certain material items?

If you are in the business of yoga, whether a studio owner, private yoga teacher, or brand CEO, I would encourage a move from thinking about only profit to liberating all, especially peoples who are oppressed. This can look like offering donation or pay-what-you-can classes, sliding scale and tiered pricing, and scholarships to certain marginalized communities and making it clear that you will support and help those unable to afford the services.

For everyone, know that how you spend your money matters. Who you invest in and buy products and services from matters. Diversify and make it a priority to support BIPOC, LGBTQIA+, and other historically marginalized teachers who are doing liberatory work. Help them flourish.

This work is about deprogramming: creating equity for one another and speaking freely and authentically. It's about putting collaboration over competition and community over individual profit, having a relationship with our ancestors and nature, and using the privilege we hold for social justice. As The Red Nation shared in their book *The Red Deal: Indigenous Action to Save Our Earth*, "Healing the planet is ultimately about creating infrastructures of caretaking that will replace infrastructures of capitalism. Capitalism is contrary to life. Caretaking promotes life."

For me, that means collaborating on all wellness-based projects so that I amplify and lift the voices of others alongside my own. It's about holding space for BIPOC-only classes, operating and teaching outside the standard yoga studio model, learning about my ancestors and connecting to Sikhism as my values model, taking sabbaticals from work to allow myself to rest, focusing on things other than making profits (and giving the middle finger to late-stage capitalism), breaking free from the rat race, and keeping up a daily sadhana (spiritual practice). I work with teachers and coaches who understand systems of oppression and don't bypass these real inequalities. I have turned down projects that didn't match my values, sometimes recommending other BIPOC teachers I felt were a better fit.

I want to offer nuance and spaciousness here. In the past, yoga teachers and devoted practitioners were monks, ascetics, and hermits from society. They didn't have the pressures we have today of making money to survive, to feed themselves and their families. Even today in India, I have seen the wandering ascetics, with their long beards and tattered orange tunics, who go to people's homes and ask for food. And people happily give them money and food. This is socially acceptable and ingrained as a part of the culture. The community comes together to provide support and meet the needs of basic living.

The conflict in the present day is that we need money to survive. Under our current unfair and rigged version of capitalism, many people are unable to keep up with the nonstop pressure to keep going. The relentless pursuit of profit at all costs has led us to this critical juncture marked by profound racial, economic, and health disparities, intertwined with the tragic challenge of climate change. We and our planet are all suffering under these conditions.

Our personal experiences, headlines, and social media regularly point to the result of this cycle—burnout, exhaustion, loneliness, stress, depression, and climate anxiety. Rising costs and lack of affordable housing, coupled with stagnant wages for working-class people, are threatening to collapse the middle class of America.

Most yoga teachers I know are not raking it in. In fact, most are making below a livable wage. I've had my fair share of money struggles as a yoga teacher and am now able to teach full-time because of community and family support around me. (This is another way to look at abundance outside of the strictly financial and to redefine wealth.) I live with my partner in his parents' (my in-laws') home and drive their 2005 van that they no longer use. This means I am not paying rent or a car payment. If I had these payments on top of student loan payments, living expenses, and the multiple trainings I take per year, I just wouldn't be able to sustain myself. I feel supported by them and know they have my back.

Most of us are operating in a late-stage capitalistic world. Even if we want to abolish the system, we are still existing within these harmful systems. Yoga teachers should be paid fairly and substantially for their knowledge, energy, service, and time. This is one reason I offer sliding scale, tiered pricing, and equity-based models for my students and clients. If someone has the means (think, people living in million-dollar homes, medium and huge corporations, and those with residual income), they should pay more.

In conversation with a fellow South Asian teacher about the financial side of yoga and how infinitely complex and nuanced it is, we both came to the same conclusion. We want teachers to keep making money teaching yoga *while* grappling with the ethics of HOW you can teach yoga from a place of love, compassion, justice, and equity and do your part to dismantle these exploitative systems.

We can survive and move past late-stage capitalism by building skills, connecting with neighbors, forming community, growing our own food (and sharing it), consuming less, and sharing our abundance with others. Wealth is not a zero-sum game. If you win, it doesn't mean I have to lose. As one of my teachers shared with me, "A rising tide lifts all boats." Free yourself from limiting beliefs that keep you in competition and comparison with others around you. We have to come together, to support and care for one another. We need one another more than ever.

We can operate differently at an individual and community level. However, this is not a replacement for the major political- and societal-level changes that are desperately needed. My hope is that if we apply some of these changes at an individual level, we will have the space, time, and energy to be part of the effort to create change at a much larger scale. Many of us are recognizing that capitalism is not capable of providing the equitable, inclusive, and sustainable future we seek.

For generations, Indigenous communities have understood that wealth and abundance are inherent in our natural ecosystems. We can similarly draw inspiration from the mushrooms and the forest, or the mycorrhizal networks, where we find examples of synergies, mutual exchange, and continuously increasing levels of abundance. I think about my ancestors in Punjab who worked with the land to grow food and care for one another.

The last time I went home to the Central Valley to visit my family, I was greeted warmly by my two aunts. My immediate family lives within twenty minutes of my four aunts and cousins. They all support and take care of one another. One day, all eleven of us went on a walk around the neighborhood. Different generations on a sunset walk. Both of my aunts work nights at Foster Farms, a poultry factory, work my mom also did for thirteen years in a row, and they both gave me money as pyar (love) before I left. Giving money in this way is a common practice in Punjabi culture. I felt tears arise because, looking in, you would think they have so little financially. However, they still know the abundance of giving. I am deeply touched by what my extended family has taught me about love, giving, and being there for one another.

For the yoga practitioner: allow yourself to become aware of when your desire is controlling you, including when your desire is directing your yoga practice. Capitalism feeds off of our attachments and desire to be happy, especially when we believe that happiness is something that is derived externally. Traditional yoga teaches us that happiness is an inside job.

Joy is innately within you. It doesn't have to be bought or earned.

8

THE NUANCES OF APPROPRIATION AND PRACTICING WITH INTEGRITY

THE CONVERSATION AROUND cultural appropriation has come to the fore since 2016. I am frequently asked to help people answer the question: *If I practice yoga, am I culturally appropriating?* To ease your mind as a fellow student and practitioner, in my opinion, you are not culturally appropriating if you practice yoga.

Cultural exchange and appreciation are beautiful and create opportunities for different groups of people to connect on a deeper level. This is necessary for healthy interpersonal relationships and fosters open-mindedness.

I know I have loved taking my close friends with me to big Punjabi weddings and seeing how thrilled they were to be able to dress in saris, eat pakoras and samosas, and (attempt to) dance giddha and bhangra on the dance floor. This is not something they would have been able to experience otherwise. Similarly, it has been an honor to be invited into medicine and plant ceremonies led by Indigenous elders and partake in something thousands of years old. Being guided by someone who has intimate ties to the culture, practice, land, and ancestry makes a huge difference.

What these examples illustrate is the importance of being *invited* to participate in these exchanges, whether they are parties, ceremonies, or other cultural practices. Someone from the culture is welcoming you in, and you, as the guest and participant, come in with respect and reverence, with a willingness to learn and be guided.

My friends didn't go to my cousin's wedding and start making fun of the customs like putting a golden paste of haldi (turmeric) all over the groom's arms, even though it was foreign to them. I didn't go into the plant and medicine ceremony and assume I knew more than these elders who invited me. I didn't believe that because I had attended one ceremony, I was now a master and could also distribute plant medicine.

In the context of respectful cultural exchange and appreciation, there is an understanding that these practices and rituals have been passed down over generations and that the culture holders have spent years learning, integrating, and studying, whether informally or formally. There is so much context around cultural customs and rituals. There is a relationship that has been built for generations between stewards of practices and those practices, the land, and spirit.

This also holds true for yoga. Yoga is deeply profound and even I, a practitioner and student for over ten years now, have only really scratched the surface of my own studies, reflection, understanding, self-exploration, and knowledge. Simply taking a 200-hour training does not make me an expert. And taking five hundred or one thousand hours of training does not take us any further to mastery.

Jnana yoga, or the yoga of wisdom or knowledge, teaches us that wisdom is a practical knowledge about how life works. And this wisdom is gleaned through attaining knowledge of the true nature of reality through study, self-inquiry, and contemplation. It is the higher awareness gleaned from life's experiences and the understanding that comes from careful examination of direct experience. This means living our yoga is applying what we are learning to our life and learning from our experiences. This is why it is important to take our yoga off the mat and into the world. To apply the teachings.

Being on the path of yoga requires humility, respect, and taking on the mindset of a student. We are lifelong students. Appropriation occurs when we disregard the teachers and practitioners before us and become arrogant.

Let's dive into a few definitions of cultural appropriation:

- When members of a dominant culture take aspects from a culture of another ethnicity or racial group they have typically oppressed and use them for personal interest or profit.
- Taking an aspect of a culture that is not one's own and using it for oneself, without regard for the context, respect, or even acknowledgment of the culture it's from.
- When individuals in positions of power or privilege commodify traditions from cultures that are not their own for the sake of fashion, trends, or profit.

Cultural appropriation can apply to anyone—not only white people. However, it is most problematic when members of a dominant culture appropriate minority cultures because the former operates as a system that inherently promotes the idea of some people being superior to others. As Michelle Cassandra Johnson lays out in her book, *Skill in Action*, this hierarchy is constructed based on various aspects of identity, including race, class, age, religion, gender, ability, and sexual orientation. It sets the standard for what is considered "normal," granting those who conform to these norms greater access to power. The dominant culture acts as a gatekeeper, deciding who can access power and navigate life with more ease. This can lead to hegemony, the forced dominance of a particular ideology or way of thinking—as in when systems favor white people while oppressing communities and people of color.

The *Dismantling Racism* workbook exposes the pervasive nature of societal biases. It highlights how society often idealizes thin, blond, white women as the standard of beauty and this bias perpetuated by media, advertising, and cultural norms can lead to body image issues, discrimination, and limited opportunities for those who don't fit this standard. This text also challenges the misconception and bias that welfare recipients are primarily Black or brown individuals lacking responsibility, while disregarding the far-reaching consequences of white-collar fraud in the business world which costs the US billions of dollars annually. Additionally, the historical and ongoing requirement for people to speak English, as imposed on Indigenous peoples and individuals from Central and South America, is a deliberate attempt to undermine community and culture.

Other examples of the dominant culture include the following:

- Cisheteronormativity: the assumption that all people are and should be cis and heterosexual. This leads to the marginalization of the LBGTQIA+ community, where structural discrimination and violence occurs against them. This leads to internalized homophobia, isolation, and other mental health issues.
- Patriarchy: a social system where men control a disproportionately large share of social, economic, political, and religious power. Women are expected to prioritize the household over careers, are paid less than men, hold fewer positions of power, and are deemed less than simply due to gender assumptions.
- Christianity: Christian values and practices are considered the norm and have played a huge role in shaping Western culture, including law, literature, celebrations, et cetera. Every other religion is seen as the other.
- Colonialism: this usually involves the colonizer forcing their views, beliefs, cultural values, and practices on the original inhabitants of the lands. An example here is the Canadian residential school system, in which the government forced Indigenous children into boarding schools, where they were stripped of their native language, religion, and practices. Many of these children were subjected to physical and sexual abuse, were forbidden from seeing their families, and had their legal identity of their tribe removed.
- Capitalism: this is the dominant economic system in the world. Its values of individualism and competitiveness have

now infiltrated our entire worldview. Capitalism has led to globalization and brought great inequalities and environmental degradation.

When talking about both dominant culture and appropriation, we also have to look at power relations. In a decolonizing wellness course I took, we looked at the forms of power. *Power Over* is the power that is exercised over others and oftentimes uses fear. And then there is positive and transformational power, *Power Within*, to believe in yourself, have hope, and take action. *Power With* means to build solidarity with others on reciprocity and love, and *Power To* is to make change and make a difference in the world.

Both in dominant culture and cultural appropriation, there is the usage of Power Over dynamics. We are not all on equal footing but hold varying degrees of power and privilege. Examples here are white women adopting Black hairstyles like cornrows and dreadlocks for fashion and "fun," while Black women are told to change their *natural* hair to look "more professional" in a work setting. Then we have sports teams that use Indigenous mascots. The National Congress of American Indians has a clear position that this is derogatory and creates a one-dimensional negative stereotype of Indigenous people. This also ignores the history of genocide and allows white people to capitalize on cultural superiority, racial tensions, and violence. Cultural appropriation causes harm to the source culture it is appropriating from.

In his groundbreaking 1978 book *Orientalism*, postcolonial studies scholar Edward Said defined Orientalism as "a style of thought based upon an ontological and epistemological distinction made between 'the Orient' and . . . 'the Occident.'" This is a created binary between the "East" and the "West," where the East is seen as foreign, primitive, chaotic, and deserving of being colonized, while the West is familiar, civilized, progressive, and logical and needs to be the one to take care of the barbaric East. This positioned Western colonial powers to take on a paternalistic role in "the Orient" because "they can't do it themselves." The West's material investment in establishing and upholding the fabrication of Orientalism sanctioned the violence of European imperialism in countries like India. This is another example of hegemony. Orientalism leads the way for further cultural appropriation, where white folks consider themselves as the authority to write the texts on behalf of the East, to appropriate spiritual symbols as their own, and more. This is how we see Western medicine as the norm and Eastern medicine as alternative. It also sets the stage for certain groups of people to be labeled as terrorists, while other groups that take the same actions are said "to be defending themselves." It creates an artificial binary where harm can be justified.

As Sonny Singh Brooklynwalla shares, "The thing about cultural appropriation is that the appropriator does not have to face the same consequences that we do for practicing our culture or faith. For them, it is an accessory that can be taken on or off at will, while for us, it is a way of life."

An example is Kundalini yoga as taught by Yogi Bhajan, whose real name is Harbhajan Singh. The practitioners of this school of yoga wear white turbans and change their names to Sikhi ones. I've been in classes and workshops where the teachers wear the white turban and don all-white clothing only to teach and then, once the class is over, they go back to their regular clothing. This feels like a costume that is put on to play the role of a Kundalini yoga teacher. Yogi Bhajan spread a diluted and whitewashed Sikhism to his followers and students, combined it with Hatha Yoga practices and techniques, and marketed it as Kundalini yoga. He characterized it as a secret ancient technology that he was sharing for the first time. Yogi Bhajan made millions of dollars, started multiple businesses, and was accused of sexual abuse by hundreds of his female students. He was an ultimate scam artist masquerading as a spiritual guru. In the Kundalini yoga training as taught by Yogi Bhajan I took in 2019, the Trataka practice was to stare into the eyes of a picture of Yogi Bhajan, and that was a huge red flag for me and something I could not participate in. I want to add nuance and complexity here. After learning about Yogi Bhajan's abuse and background, I felt I could no longer teach Kundalini Yoga with a clear conscience. However, the year-long training led by Siri Bahadur Khalsa, Mehtab Benton, and Steph

"Navjeet" Smith was a transformative experience for me. The long practices focused on kriyas, mantras and meditation, lifestyle recommendations, and anchoring back into the tenets of Sikhism rang true for me. There are large aspects of this training that I still use and live by today.

Most of the elder men in my family—both my grandfathers and my uncles, as well as my younger cousins—wear a turban, or what is known as a *dastar* or *pag* in Panjabi. A turban is worn by both Sikh men and women to represent their faith, to showcase their connection to Sikhism. It also represents equality, honor, spirituality, self-respect, and piety.

After 9/11, many Sikhs faced harassment, assault, and violence by Americans who confused them with terrorists and were acting out of Islamophobia. My grandfather, who had worn a turban for seventy years at that point, felt obligated to remove it due to the threat of violence and instead wore a baseball cap. For him, his turban was not a costume he wore to play the part of a Sikhi follower: it was who he is. And due to the threat of violence, he was forced to remove it.

That is a big difference when we look at cultural appropriation. For others, it gets to be an accessory that is removed at will. However, for those from the culture, it is a part of who they are and something that can expose them to marginalization.

Another example of this is the Dotbusters, a Hinduphobic New Jersey hate group primarily made up of white men, which attacked Indian Americans from 1975 to 1993. They called themselves the Dotbusters, referring to the bindis that primarily South Asian women wear on the center of their forehead between the eyebrows. This hate group came out with a letter in 1987, detailing how they would terrorize Indian Americans: "We are an organization called the Dotbusters. We have been around for 2 [sic] years. We will go to any extreme to get Indians to move out of Jersey City. If I'm walking down the street and I see a Hindu and the setting is right, I will hit him or her." Indians and Indian Americans were attacked, beaten, and even killed by this hate group.

Now consider the people not of South Asian descent who wear bindis as a fashion accessory to music festivals. For them, the bindi becomes a fun thing to wear. It is not something these attendees are worried is going to get them attacked or killed. They are wearing these bindis as a cute accessory, without taking into account the history behind them and the real reason people from the source culture wear them. This is appropriation.

Researcher and Professor Amanda Lucia, in her book *White Utopias*, explores festivals like Burning Man and Lightning in a Bottle and how it is usually white people who participate in religious exoticism by adopting Indigenous and Indic spiritualities while attending them. These festivals can become an exclusive space where anything goes and where appropriation is rampant. As someone who enjoys attending and teaching at transformational festivals, I've found them to be vibrant spaces for connection, creativity, and self-expression. However, I also recognize that these spaces often unintentionally perpetuate forms of cultural appropriation and spiritual exoticism that conflict with the deeper traditions of yoga and other non-Western spiritual practices. I believe there is great potential for these festivals to evolve into spaces that celebrate cultural diversity while honoring the origins of the spiritual practices they highlight. With greater awareness and intentionality, these events could become better platforms for healing, education, and authentic cross-cultural engagement. This could involve inviting teachers from source cultures to lead workshops and rituals with proper cultural context, welcoming Indigenous leaders as equal partners, and practicing responsible environmental stewardship by aligning the festival with sustainable practices that honor the land. This genuine dialogue and collaboration are needed.

Let's go over some specific examples of how cultural appropriation can show up in the yoga space.

Not Acknowledging the Roots of Yoga

I was a guest on a podcast in 2020, and one of the interviewers shared that they had recently learned that yoga comes from South Asia. She is not the only person I have come across who has become aware of this fundamental fact after years of practicing. Nothing about the yoga they had experienced suggested to them it was anything but a modern fitness class at best and a white woman's sport at worst. At least this interviewer was happy to acknowledge this fact once she learned it.

Gwyneth Paltrow, founder of Goop, took heat in 2018 for taking credit for yoga becoming popular. She said in an interview with *WSJ Magazine*:

> *I remember when I started doing yoga and people were like, "What is yoga? She's a witch. She's a freak."*
>
> *Forgive me if this comes out wrong . . . but I went to do a yoga class in L.A. recently and the 22-year-old girl behind the counter was like, "Have you ever done yoga before?" And literally I turned to my friend, and I was like, "You have this job because I've done yoga before."*

It is important for us as yoga practitioners to acknowledge the roots, history, and teachings of yoga as sacred wisdom. We need to recognize the source culture, to educate ourselves and continue learning, and to research. Otherwise, we just make it up as we go along, which distorts the truth over time. We have to acknowledge the brown and Black people who were the original stewards of this path and practice.

Goop is just one of the many big brands that appropriate and profit from yoga. CorePower, Lululemon, the list goes on.

Making a Profit or Turning Yoga into a Business Without Any Credit or Acknowledgment to the Culture or Indigenous Peoples

When I see statements like the ones on CorePower's website (see pg. 79), which include words like "found," "found an opportunity," "discovered," "make yoga convenient," and "new yoga," my guard comes up. Particularly the "new yoga" statement. Nowhere on the website is there an acknowledgment of where yoga originated.

Studios like CorePower and other chain companies churn out hundreds of yoga teachers a year who have been taught to learn and memorize a script for their version of an asana (primarily vinyasa) class, in which the spiritual and historical aspects are stripped out. These hopeful, aspiring yoga teachers come in with good intentions, but due to the negligence of companies that commodify yoga for profit, people lose out on all that is available to them through the holistic understanding of yoga.

This commercialization of yoga teacher trainings, which are often cash cows for yoga studios and help them stay open, produce inadequately trained instructors who have been trained in asana only. As will be discussed in an upcoming chapter, there are 200-hour yoga teacher trainings that don't have any history or philosophy at all. However, these trainings do include modules on the business of being a yoga teacher, how to market yourself using social media, and more.

These pressures to cater yoga to market demands lead to misrepresentations and distortions of yoga practices, perpetuating cultural appropriation. Yoga studios and brands that emphasize profit margins may also prioritize class sizes, focusing on quantity over quality. They diminish the importance of individual attention, personal connection, and supportive community spaces. Sangha, or community, is an important part of being on the spiritual path of yoga. And of course, as previously discussed, there is the total disregard for the lineage and heritage of yoga as an ancient practice of wisdom.

There are many examples of how this plays out: "Nama-stay-in-bed" tank tops, the proliferation of expensive yoga mats and yoga pants, inaccessible class and retreat costs, and signs that read "No Sanskrit here" in yoga studios to appeal to a wider audience.

In making profit-driven motives the priority, the essence, integrity, and inclusive nature of yoga is compromised. And this applies for all traditions and businesses. When profit is prioritized over people and care for the planet and each other, we all suffer as a result.

Unwilling to Understand the True Goals and Intentions of Yoga

Remember my story about the woman who wanted to work with me privately but only for the physical benefits of yoga asana? She didn't even want to hear about how yoga is a practice and path rooted in spirituality and philosophy. This is someone who simply did not care to know. I don't think everyone who practices yoga has to practice only for spiritual reasons and to study the philosophy. If you want to practice yoga asana only, sure, go ahead! That might be where you are in your journey with yoga, and that is completely fine. However, can you be open to knowing there is more to yoga and acknowledging that truth?

I encourage students and practitioners to be open-minded. To be willing to understand why yoga was founded. This is a path designed to help us out of our suffering (dukkha) and toward moksha (liberation). It is a path of self-realization and transformation that may take lifetime(s). This is one big reason we do not need to rush as yoga students and teachers. Take your time studying, reflecting, unlearning, integrating, and self-adjusting. Our yoga is meant to be lived and understood in every aspect of our life.

Thousands of years ago, these yogis and sages took the time to understand the depths of their minds and left us with knowledge and wisdom. I have great respect for the texts that hold the wisdom of our ancestors who took time to figure this stuff out and codify it. It is a travesty to erase, disregard, and dilute all they left to us.

I encourage students and practitioners to learn the philosophy and really understand their intentions for being on this path of yoga. For what purpose are you practicing and studying? At the mental health center where I teach, one of the students asked me, "You always speak about intention. Is it really that important?" And to that student, and to you, I say—*yes*!

Sankalpa is our conscious way to focus our determination and resolve, to set an intention with meaning. To align ourselves to an affirmation, decision, choice, or guiding principle or value that is our compass and guiding light. Exploring our intention also gets us to self-inquire and reflect. To understand ourselves more deeply.

The purpose of sankalpa can be summarized by Katha Upanishad Chapter 1, Section 3 Verse 14: "*uttiṣṭhata jāgrata prāpya varānnibodhata.*" This means "Get up, wake up (arise), and stop not until the goal is realized!" Our sankalpa is a lifelong and sincere commitment, something we come back to daily, every time we become aware again, and with every breath. A reflection question here is, What are you committed to?

In modern yoga, the goals for many have shifted. This can be linked to treating yoga as:

- medicine
- a fitness regime
- physical therapy and rehab
- a mind–body practice
- stress reduction and relaxation
- psychological treatment (e.g., somatic therapy)
- the subject of neuroscientific and scientific studies

Overall, this is all positive because it creates more opportunities for people to gain the benefits of yoga. However, the other side is that classical yoga gets stripped out, and the goals get changed. This is not to say goals like stress reduction and healing trauma are wrong. The point is that it is possible to pursue these new goals of yoga while still respecting its roots.

Although yoga is being treated as a healing system and a complementary therapy and being recommended by doctors to their patients, it is still not covered under insurance. Changing this would make it accessible for more people. There have been hundreds of studies proving yoga is helpful in treating pain, depression, anxiety, and trauma, but still it is considered an "alternative healing method." If we are going to view yoga as a physical and mental healing modality under its medicalization, we should then at least make it accessible to more people and compensate facilitators and teachers.

I think about Jon Kabat-Zinn founding Mindfulness-Based Stress Reduction (MBSR), which was a brand he created after studying Buddhism. Zinn is quoted as saying, "I bent over backward to avoid being seen as Buddhist, New Age, or plain flaky." To be seen as scientifically credible in the 1970s, he wiped out the Eastern roots to make the brand completely secular and more legitimate in the eyes of other professionals. And it worked. MBSR has made mindfulness incredibly popular. This knowledge seems to ascribe more value when it is presented by a white man. However, mindfulness (Samma sati) is only one part of Buddhism's Eightfold Path, and one part of this path to live a noble and moral life. A tool used to help discern from "skillful" and "unskillful" behavior, not only to reduce personal stress. In Western secularization, the roots and ultimate goal get erased.

Another example is the Western medical community renaming the pranayama practice of anuloma viloma or nadi shodhana (alternate nostril breathing) as cardiac coherence breathing. Why was this necessary? Anuloma viloma or nadi shodhana already has an English name! Colonizers time and time again have tried to wipe out our ancestral and intuitive knowledge. This information did not exist in Western science before it was introduced from BIPOC traditions and healing systems.

Decontextualizing

This brings us to *decontextualizing*, the act of removing or separating something from its original context or setting. It involves isolating a particular element, statement, concept, or object from the circumstances, background, or environment in which it was originally intended to be understood. When something is decontextualized, its meaning, significance, or interpretation may change or become ambiguous due to the absence of the original context. This process occurs in yoga in many different ways.

Some examples of this include the emergence of classes like beer yoga and goat yoga. What do beer or goats have to do with yoga? Beer is antithetical to the path of yoga in that alcohol clouds our perspective, while yoga seeks to bring clarity. Goats are brought in for a sense of entertainment and marketing appeal, but yoga is not about entertainment. *In fact, being bored or restless in a yoga class or in your own practice is a good thing.* You get an opportunity to observe the boredom and restlessness and see how that shows up for you. When boredom arises, what is your next tendency? To immediately seek sensation in the form of your phone, TV, gossip, or something else? Can you sit with your boredom and be with it? Learn from it? In fact, being with boredom actually leads to creative thinking. I would encourage us to not stifle this natural brilliance within us by turning to external sensation all the time.

Another way decontextualization shows up is in changing tones of mantras or not taking the time to learn how to chant correctly. A mantra is a word or phrase chosen to represent a particular aspect of reality. Repeating a mantra helps us concentrate and direct our energy toward that concept. For mantra, pronounced "mun-tra" in Sanskrit, it is important to chant them correctly. The pronunciation, tone, understanding of chandas or metrics, and pauses make a big difference. Sanskrit, literally meaning "well-constructed" (samskṛta), boasts a precise pronunciation system. This deliberate design allows proper pronunciation to unlock deeper layers of meaning beyond the surface definitions of words. Anyone who uses mantras or Sanskrit should endeavor to learn how to use it properly. I acknowledge that many yoga trainings do not spend any or enough time to help students learn Sanskrit. Even all of the trainings I have done have not focused on this. This has impacted my own pronunciation of Sanskrit words, where I, too, have work to do on improving. May we learn without being ashamed of our current starting position! We all have to start from somewhere.

Dilution can also occur when we mistake Patanjali's eight limbs of yoga as the only path or entirety of yoga or when we think of Sanskrit as the only language of yoga. There are many other systems in yoga that work with other limbs (angas), like the similar Noble Eightfold Path of Buddhism; the Goraksha Shataka, an early Hatha Yoga text with six limbs; the seven limbs of the Mrgendratantra and Gheranda Samhita; or the fifteen of the Aparokshanubhuti. Within yoga, there are other ideologies and schools of thought beyond Patanjali's eight-limbed path, such as Hatha Yoga, Bhakti yoga, Buddhist yoga, Tantra yoga, and Laya yoga. There will be more than we will ever be able to know, study, and practice.

Modern India is incredibly diverse, with twenty-two official languages, 122 major languages, and over 19,500 dialects, most of which are hundreds or even thousands of years old. It is true that the Yoga Sutras, Bhagavad Gita, Vedas, Upanishads, and Itihasa Purana were written in Sanskrit; however, the Epics, the Puranas, the Bhagavad Gita, and other yogic, religious, and spiritual texts were translated to regional languages to make them accessible to folks who didn't have access to Sanskrit due to caste, religion, gender, and socioeconomic factors. This also coincided with the Bhakti movement (sixth or seventh century CE), which helped uplift the most marginalized members of Indian society and played a key role in the development of vernacular literature. Gautama Buddha chose to give sermons not in Sanskrit, the language of the elite, but in the local language of Magadhu Prakrit, to reach more people and to make it accessible. His teachings were also written in Pali and not in Sanskrit. Thus, we can say that Sanskrit is *one* of the languages of yoga so as not to miss out on all the vernacular spiritual literature.

This decontextualization can also occur when we dumb down things in yoga or do not take the time to understand context or purpose. In our modern time, we practice Savasana at the end of the class to allow the body to relax, to rest, and to integrate. Ancient yogis practiced Savasana as a way to relax the body and mind as well. These benefits are mentioned in texts like the Hatha Yoga Pradipika and the Gheranda Samhita. However, there is more to the story here. Why does Savasana mean *Corpse* or *Death Pose*? Savasana was traditionally practiced as a dissolution meditation, as a way to dissolve the body and unite with the divine. To lose ourselves as the actor and to realize that there is more than the body and mind. In yoga, a conscious death represents the transition from human life to eternity. Savasana also reminds us that the cycle of birth–life–death is always around us and a part of us. Something I teach my students is that we can always begin anew.

A quote from Daniel Simpson's *The Truth of Yoga* brings this discussion together:

> *Everyone is free to create a new version of yoga philosophy. However, it seems wise to engage with tradition before going freestyle. The alternative is like trying to play jazz with no knowledge of scales or trying to paint abstract art without learning to draw. We might well be gifted with insight, but the chances of making a mess are considerably higher.*

***

When folks worry about the cultural appropriation of yoga, they are oftentimes looking for a checklist. Should I say *namaste* at the end of the class? Should I use Sanskrit while teaching asana? However, the real inquiry lies in understanding the roots, theories, and histories so that we can see how cultural appropriation happens as a result of colonialism, oppression, and Orientalism.

One antidote to cultural appropriation is cultural *appreciation* of the kind I laid out at the beginning of the chapter. This means taking the time to learn and be a lifelong student, showing respect and reverence, honoring the culture and people, and crediting cultural practices from other cultures. It means being willing to try to understand and admitting when you are wrong or have caused harm, whether unintentionally or intentionally. It is also means admitting when you do not know something or don't even have enough context to understand it.

The first step to knowing something is to admit you don't know it!

I love Thich Nhat Hanh practice of asking the simple question *You think so?* He recommends this question as a great way to check in with your perceptions and to wade through layers of views, beliefs, opinions, and attitudes to see what is actually true. He has said that 99 percent of our perceptions are incorrect. And I agree with that through my own personal experience. I have been shocked time and time again (and humored) when a thought or perception I had is entirely false. And now I let this wisdom help me be less rigid in my beliefs. By not being so rigid, I am able to accept myself and others with more understanding. We all have our own lived experiences and perspectives that affect how we view the world. A part of this practice of *You think so?* eliminates the need for our ego to be right and for our perceptions to be set in stone. We can accept being wrong and can be willing to change our views.

A way to practice this self-inquiry is to notice when you have a thought about something—it could be a negative thought about yourself or a belief you hold about the world. At this point, take a deep breath, adopt an attitude of compassionate curiosity, and ask yourself, *You think so?* Listen and see what comes up. Why do you have that belief? Did anything change?

This practice is something I try daily and teach in my classes. This practice is a gentle way to catch ourselves and stay open. To know our perceptions are often incorrect doesn't make us bad people. It means we are human.

If you believe you know something about a cultural practice that is not your own, ask yourself, *You think so?* Then course correct.

We have to let go of any shame around not knowing something. Not knowing only means that now there is room to learn and grow. We can also all get better at admitting when we are wrong or have changed our minds! To allow new information and learning to yield and release thoughts and beliefs that you once considered immovable. This is the beauty of being human: knowing that we are all capable of changing and growing.

Here's an example of my own learning and growth: From 2021 to 2022, I worked with and taught yoga to autistic children. I found myself alternating between the terms *autistic kids* and *kids with autism* when referencing this work. After collaborating with an agency on a video about how to honor the roots of yoga, the organization informed me that it had to remove the last slide due to concerns about the language used. My reference to kids with autism in the video was flagged. After getting feedback and researching, the agency learned that the autistic community prefers the term *autistic kids*. I remember receiving that email and noticing my body feeling hot. A sense of *Oh no, I did something wrong* rose in me. I took a short walk outside to regulate myself, and in that moment, I spoke kindly to myself. I said, "It's okay, you did not know, my love. However, now you have learned something. How wonderful. Now you know which term is preferred and what to use." I came back to the email in a more regulated state and expressed my gratitude to the sender for bringing this to my attention.

I remind my students, especially the teenagers, that we are going to make mistakes all the time. We do not need to shame ourselves. What counts is how we choose to respond, to take the learning and move forward with greater understanding. To take accountability and own up. This moves us from denial to greater self-acceptance.

In this same way, I truly believe students want to practice with more respect and to honor the source culture. To have more understanding. To practice cultural appreciation rather than cultural appropriation.

At a music and yoga festival where I presented a decolonizing yoga panel, a white student told me that her friends were making fun of her for wanting to attend. But she didn't give in to their perspective. She simply walked away to my panel, calling over her shoulder, "Bye! I'm going to learn how to be a better white person!"

This made me laugh. I admire her. I admire all people who want to become better and can admit they have room to grow.

9

THE EROSION OF SPIRITUAL AND CULTURAL FOUNDATIONS

ONE WAY THAT colonialism in the history of yoga still shows up today is in the whitewashing of many yoga spaces and how yoga is practiced in those spaces.

I experienced this whitewashing in a major way at a yoga and music festival where I led a decolonizing yoga panel. After the panel, my friend and I were making our way through the festival grounds when a white woman stopped me.

"I was at the decolonizing yoga panel where you spoke!"

I smiled and waited for her to continue. Several others had shared positive feedback, so I thought this woman was about to say something positive as well.

"All I wanted to say is, the yoga studios . . . us white people, it's all we have."

The smile on my face froze as I tried to figure out what direction this conversation was about to head in.

"And the asana, it's an entry point for so many people. Why is that bad? The physical practice allows so many people to find yoga and spirituality."

As she spoke, I noticed that she was holding a glass of beer and was ever so slightly swaying from side to side.

I took a beat before responding, "No one is saying to take the yoga studios and asana away! We are highlighting the lack of diversity and how yoga studios, which are primarily owned and run by white people, can do better. To move from teaching yoga as a self-serving individualistic pursuit to one that emphasizes our interconnectedness.

The way yoga is taught in the studio's cherry picks out certain elements of yoga as pacifying techniques and ostracizes people of color who want to learn yoga to find freedom, and some of that freedom has to come through systemic change."

"There is nothing wrong with only practicing the physical practice and it being led by white people," she replied. "That's all I'm going to say."

I felt my frustration rising, but I tried to remain composed, neutral, and compassionate. I took a breath and decided to remain open and receptive. I recognized that this woman is not the only person to feel this way.

"Thank you for sharing your perspective," I said to her. "But it does sound like perhaps you are not wanting to understand the perspective we shared during the panel? No one wants to take anything away from you. As the first step, it is about expanding the practice to include more of yoga and bring in BIPOC who have long felt excluded from their own ancestral and cultural practices."

She looked at me with anger. "You don't have to take that tone. There is no need for things to get aggressive. I just wanted to share my perspective."

This story is a prime example of white fragility and tone policing. I had wanted to encourage this person to realize that the "entryway" that she spoke of has become the destination for most modern practitioners. It is fitness for fitness's sake, for aesthetic and vanity purposes. It has become another tool of white supremacy. As Aarti Inamdar shared in her Instagram post, "To decolonize yoga includes recognizing that these practices are tied to a culture and people. When we pull the practices out of context as a fitness trend, we devalue the culture of origin, the practice, and the people."

While researching this book, I was astounded to see that the vast majority of books about yoga that I came across were written by white people. Why are white people seen as the experts and figureheads within the yogic space, when the knowledge they present is actually, at best, borrowed and, in reality, mostly appropriated from other cultures? Professor Amanda Lucia writes, "What began as a quest for authentic roots ends up consuming them and reproducing them through the perspectival lens of the white subject. **It becomes another moment of what the Australian Aboriginal scholar Aileen Moreton-Robinson calls white possessivism, the seemingly ubiquitous expression of white claims to access and entitlement.**"

White folks take yoga on as their own without building relationships or giving credit. They create their own exclusive communities that are present across yoga festivals, yoga trainings, and yoga organizations. When white voices are promoted as the authorities in the yoga space, there is also a sanitization and sterilization that happens widely in yoga classes and spaces. This is what occurs when folks from the original culture are dismissed, not brought in, or disregarded. Once the teachings have been co-opted, where is the need for the original stewards of the practices, culture, and lands from which they come?

Yoga as a Prescriptive Model

This is the harmful path of erasure, which in this context, is the ongoing marginalization, appropriation, and exclusion of certain cultural practices, lineages, and voices within the broader yoga community.

I see this in the way the mental health and healing community has co-opted yoga. Yoga has been forced through the same Eurocentric treatment that the mental health therapy industry has in America: sanitized, offered as a one-size-fits-all solution, and focused on "treating" the illness instead of looking at the person as a whole, bypassing the larger systems that cause people to be unwell *and to stay unwell.*

One of my peers in the yoga space privately shared with me how, during a trauma-informed yoga teacher training that she took, participants were advised to create space between them and their students, or "clients." They were told to keep sessions within the confines of the time offered, to not talk about themselves, and to not build a personal relationship with the client. This falls within the Eurocentric way of conducting therapy: be a "blank slate," keep it strictly professional, don't have anything personal in your office. However, in many cultures across the world, and in my experiences with my own teachers, the healer and teacher build a more intimate relationship and might share from personal experience where it can be supportive to do so. We deserve to build and access caring and authentic relationships with those we help and with those who help us.

Why are we teaching people to become more like robots and create more separation under the guise of professionalism? I think of one of my private yoga students, Archana, who has now become a dear and close friend. She initially reached out to me because she was uncomfortable with the whitewashing and appropriation she saw in local yoga studios and wanted to learn from a South Asian person instead. We spent over a year building a trusting relationship where we got to truly know one another. I think of my other private yoga student, Dalita, who I first supported through her fourth pregnancy and have since continued to see weekly at her house for over two years now. Every time I travel, I always bring her back a gift. Upon receiving one gift—a pashmina scarf from Punjab—she teared up and shared, "In Armenia, everyone would always give each other gifts and show one another how much the other person meant to them. Now here in America, no one gives gifts or shows love. We're all separated in our own homes with no coming together. You remind me of home." I too teared up.

One of my yoga teachers stays at his students' homes when he travels globally to teach yoga. This traditional teacher–student yoga relationship transcends Eurocentric-created boundaries and distance. Traditionally, students study with their teacher for decades, are guided through life's challenges and obstacles and come together in celebration. I worry that the Western mental therapy approach risks diminishing the potential of the closeness of these relationships.

I feel this pressure when I teach trauma-informed yoga to teens at mental health centers. One of the centers I worked at had a change in program director. The first program director gave me freedom in how I held space, where I was able to tailor my teaching based on the students' needs and offer options. Sure, we did yoga asana and pranayama, and I spoke about nervous system regulation as they expected, but I also brought in sound bowls for sound healing. We practiced restorative yoga asana and longer Savasana when I noticed the kids looked exhausted, which they often were, as a result of the medication they were prescribed, the constant need to be "better," and pressures of Western ways of being—the pressures of trying to keep up in school, extracurriculars, and social media comparison. I always gave students an option: you can participate or rest. We practiced creative writing exercises where I encouraged the students to reimagine a more supportive, kinder world. We spoke about what causes they cared about and what change they wished to see. Students spoke about gender equality, colonialism, animal protection, the prison industrial complex, and more. I invited students to shake their bodies and move in silly ways.

Once the second director took over the organization, things changed. Upon the completion of a restorative yoga asana session where a student remarked, "Wow, that's the best sleep I've gotten in three months!", the director called me into her office.

"Why were the kids sleeping?" she asked me.

Caught off guard, I responded, "Oh, that's restorative yoga, where poses are held for longer periods of time in supported positions to allow for deep rest. And then some students didn't want to participate, so I let them sleep using the blankets and bolsters."

She wrinkled her nose slightly and gave a small laugh. "We need to make sure students are actually learning something, not just sleeping." Completely stunned, I just nodded and left.

Yoga is fundamentally about deep rest, something that I believe we all need more of. Collectively we are all burdened, overworked, and exhausted by the pressures of trying to keep up in this late-stage capitalistic world driven by colonial violence and historical trauma. We need space to just be. Practices like Savasana and Yoga Nidra offer us that space.

The next week, one of the therapists at the same center shared with me how she was practicing hot yoga now at a studio and how much she was enjoying the challenge of the poses. I smiled and said, "Wow, that's amazing, good for you!" The next week, the program director called me into her office and shared they wanted something "more fitness-y" for the students. I was able to respond, "We do yoga asana when it is appropriate for students, and it is not every single time. I don't force students, only encourage, and I care about consent and autonomy. And yoga is more than fitness!" Her response was: "Well, that's what we want." Again I just nodded, at a loss for words. The following week, I was unceremoniously let go from that center and from my teaching position via email. It was a punch to the gut.

What I hope this story illustrates is how yoga has been reduced to a fitness fad, which means that those of us who teach it in its fullness are sidelined. Yoga's sanitization hurts those that need a deeper healing. Trauma is not a one-time occurrence. Colonial wounding, racism and intergenerational trauma require a more substantive response than the one being presented, where the modern yoga industry prefers to skirt over the causes and merely address superficial needs.

When I teach in these spaces and in the Yoga for Anxiety course I run, I speak to these deeper systemic issues and anxiety that results from forced or assimilated disconnection through colonialism. We cannot erase these histories—our bodies and nervous systems bear the brunt of what has happened. Psychologist Eduardo Duran, of Apache, Tewa, and Lakota descent, refers to this as the "soul wound," the spiritual damage that colonized and enslaved people suffer from generations of trauma. We might not have the words to express it just yet, but there are physical, mental, and emotional signs of distress. Yoga cannot be offered like a prescription the same way medicines are doled out. The individual and their story need to be taken into account and deliberate space created to offer reconnection.

Sanitization of Yoga

The sanitization of yoga has been a topic of debate and controversy. Some argue that it erodes the spiritual and cultural foundations of the practice. Others, argue that it makes yoga more accessible and inclusive. But accessible and inclusive to whom? As it stands, the sanitized version of yoga serves the dominant culture.

This sterilization of yoga also happens when certain components that make the practice seem "too ethnic" or "too other" get removed. These components can include Sanskrit, om, chanting, mantras, philosophy, and history—all things that many of us want to bring back into the space.

Yoga has been decontextualized through mockery of its rigid constraints. For example, the manifesto of yoga studio Fierce Grace proclaimed "We won't Om you" and assured people on its website that "This is not an Indian Secret Mystery Club."

A student of mine was once brought into a yoga studio as a teacher because the studio owners wanted her to teach yoga in a way that honors the roots. However, when she began questioning certain aspects of the studio—like why she was the only South Asian person on the teaching team and why there was an om poster in the bathroom—and wanted to change class names to more accurately reflect what she wanted to teach (e.g., calling it *pranayama* instead of a *breathwork class*), the studio owner pushed back and didn't want to engage in a conversation. One response the studio owner had was "My husband is Indian, and he said it's fine to have the om poster in the bathroom." There is quite a bit of cognitive dissonance here between what is being asked and then being allowed. This fits with my own experience of people and organizations saying they want to change, but then their actions do not match up with their words. A seat at the table is given with the underlying message that you are here for aesthetics, not for real change. Play the part, but don't expect to be listened to. This says, *We have no intention of sharing power with you.*

There is a reason I started working for myself and building solidarity with others who shared my values. I saw how folks in seats of authority and privilege continued to use their power as a weapon to silence and oppress. I wish to be in solidarity with those to whom I do not have to explain my humanity, where I am heard and truly understood. I am interested in seeing folks of the global majority be free—this is my path in this life. As Dalia Kinsey shared in *Decolonizing Wellness*, "Life is too short to exist in spaces that simply tolerate you." I want to be in spaces and in cocreation with others who want the same goals of reciprocal love, joy, compassion, and wild imagination for one another.

The peer who shared with me about the trauma-informed teacher training also expressed how the white teacher trainers explicitly taught the students not to use Sanskrit, mantras, chanting, or philosophy in their classes when they became teachers. The teachers leading the training felt that using these components in classes would be alienating or isolating to those with trauma. Never mind how the *erasure* of the wholeness of yoga in a yoga space would feel to South Asian yoga students with generational trauma of colonialism!

Teachers like this white trainer are being shortsighted. It doesn't help anyone to remove Sanskrit, chanting, mantras, or other traditional parts of the yoga path completely because you feel that students aren't capable of understanding or receiving them. There should at least be an acknowledgment of what isn't being taught so that students can learn on their own if they wish.

My friend ended up speaking with the owner and teacher trainers. Sadly, she was met with tons of resistance and no attempt at understanding her view.

She shared with me, "The way they were leading the training didn't sit right with me. It didn't address the harm and trauma of colonized folks having their spiritual and ancestral practices being altered for white comfort. To this day, I teach in a community center with folks who are often unhoused and have faced incredible trauma. Time and time again they tell me that the mantras and kriyas are some of the most grounding aspects of the practice. And when I teach a Sanskrit mantra, it always comes with the context of what the words mean. I think too many trauma-informed teachers underestimate what traumatized folks need to feel safe. It's better to just ask and communicate than deny them access to practices they might actually really find support the nervous system."

When open dialogue isn't encouraged, there isn't room for brave conversations or authentic relationships. When we continually sanitize and alter spiritual practices for the comfort of white people, the people from the original culture continue to be harmed and traumatized. **Whose safety are we then prioritizing in these trainings and spaces?**

In trauma-informed trainings, we often speak about giving students ample options and inviting them into practice. Autonomy and consent are centered. When we do not offer the entirety of yoga, we limit those choices and mistakenly present the view that there is a one-size-fits-all solution.

For teachers in this space, I encourage you to contextualize your offerings in terms of yoga's history and complexity. Understand the setting and who is in the room. Build trust with your students, build personal relationships, and bring in more aspects of the yoga practice. You can even ask your students if they would like to learn about yogic philosophy, if they want to practice a certain pranayama or chant.

There is a reason I worked at yoga studios for only the first six months of my teaching career. I saw very early on that teaching the way that I wanted—teaching the heart of yoga and including all components—wasn't welcome.

In the six years since I set out alone, I have taught at community centers, rehabs, foster homes, autism centers, mental health centers for teens, and private clients' homes—spaces where there isn't always so much rigidity. And I've found that I've had the most impact with my students when I have included pranayama, om chanting, philosophy, the history of yoga, and the goals for practice, and looked at colonial sources of disconnection. When practice was tailored for their individual needs.

When speaking about purusha and prakriti at a rehab center, one of my students started crying. These concepts refer to the cosmic material, and spirit or conscious energy that is at the root of all living beings. For some, these concepts can reassure us that our core essence remains good and holy, no matter what we've done in the past. That there is always time to begin again. When I asked the student who cried what this discussion was bringing up for her, she replied, "I've never had anyone tell me that I am a good person before. Because I have made poor decisions in the past and done some bad things, that became my label as a bad person. You sharing about creating that space and saying that I did a bad thing but I am not a bad person changed something for me forever."

An asana-only practice can be more alienating than one that incorporates a broader understanding of yoga. When teaching at a mental health center, I observed that some students were uninterested or unable to sit through a forty-five- to sixty-minute pure asana class. But when I introduced concepts like the mudras, the yamas, and the niyamas, along with pranayama practices, meditation, Yoga Nidra, and much longer Savasana times, they perked up.

In one session, the four kids in the group were reviewing a mudra sheet I had created for them, and they wanted to practice gyan mudra. Over the next few weeks, two of the kids came up to me and told me they were still practicing gyan mudra and meditating for a minute every morning and that this was helping them.

This clearly indicates that people want to learn and want to go deeper. We are doing a disservice to our students when we don't at least acknowledge all that there is to yoga. It could be as simple as telling a class that you will be focusing on, for example, asana, explaining why, and reminding students that there is so much more to yoga.

Why should we assume that trauma survivors can't handle the fact that yoga does not emerge from mainstream white culture? This assumption is teaching down to students. Instead, we can teach *up* to students from a place of understanding that most people like to learn.

If people don't get to learn about the other aspects of yoga, we will produce another generation that believes yoga equals asana as solely exercise. As teachers, it is our responsibility to continue to expand our perspective and acknowledge different lived experiences.

10

IS TWO HUNDRED HOURS ENOUGH?

On the Problems of Yoga Teacher Training

IT'S NOT DIFFICULT to become a certified yoga teacher in America. You might have friends or acquaintances who have become yoga teachers as a side gig, or you might have considered becoming a yoga teacher yourself. The trend suggests that to become an "authority" on yoga, a complex tradition with thousands of years of history, you only need to take a 200-hour yoga teacher training (YTT).

The credentialing body for 200-hour YTTs in the United States is the Yoga Alliance, which was created twenty-four years ago as a "voluntary registry to recognize yoga schools and yoga teachers whose training met their existing standards." It's also worth noting that yoga erupted as an industry around the time fitness was erupting as well.

It sets standards and requirements by which trainings are registered. Of the total two hundred hours, the alliance requires only thirty hours are deemed necessary for history, philosophy, and ethics. That's only 15 percent of the total training! The majority of the hours, about 155 hours, are allocated to the techniques of practice—asana, pranayama, meditation, anatomy, physiology, teaching methodology, and professional development. 60 percent of the hours are devoted to asana and sequencing of poses alone.

Other countries have different governing bodies and different requirements for YTT. I did my first teacher training in Australia, where the governing body is Yoga Australia, and the standard is a 350-hour teacher training. While the total number of hours is greater than in America, the way these hours are allocated largely toward asana is identical.

Some YTTs I've seen don't include philosophy or history at all! Some of them included things like Taoism, which isn't really related to yoga—why are trainings blending philosophies? I find this confuses students more and perpetuates the idea that all Eastern philosophies are the same. It's no wonder that the popular understanding of yoga is so reductive.

Students should be learning the foundations of yoga before going into such in-depth study of the specific techniques and tools. This grounding helps to inform practitioners and students of the holistic goals of yoga and makes it possible to apply the teachings to life—because yoga is meant to be *lived*, not just practiced for a short period of time.

Yoga studios are the primary way new yoga teachers are "produced" today—and it is effectively a production line underpinned by a capitalistic business imperative that places profit margins at the forefront. Many studios run YTTs because they are moneymakers for the studio. These trainings cost anywhere from $1,000 to over $5,000 per student. I have also seen trainings where the teacher has been studying and practicing yoga for only two years. A desire to make money, I find, can make people cut corners and rush the process. I've seen 200-hour YTTs that could be completed in as little as fourteen days. That's not enough time. As a result, unqualified teachers are pumped out.

Oftentimes, a studio will have one to four trainings a year, with about ten to thirty students in each. According to some measures, there are roughly forty-nine thousand yoga and Pilates studios in the US. Say 25 percent of those are running two trainings a year with an average of fifteen students in them each. That means there are 367,500 new yoga teachers being produced every year, who go on to teach their limited view. This means that over time, the history, philosophy, and ethics of the practice get sidelined. Meanwhile, the idea that yoga is merely exercise is perpetuated and accepted as fact.

As these new teachers are pumped out, there is also a push for these teachers to brand themselves, to stand out, and to commodify themselves. I have felt that conflict as a yoga teacher myself, feeling like I needed to promote myself to reach students and organizations to partner with and hire me.

One easy change I would encourage is requiring more of those hours to be about learning history, philosophy, and ethics. Fifteen percent is not enough. If we are to do a better job of educating yoga teachers and practitioners, we need take a more considered approach. Different yoga traditions were influenced by social, economic, political, and then later, religious influences in South Asia. It is important to keep this history and these multiple narratives alive for future generations, especially as history is being actively and purposefully erased in our current political moment.

I had an opportunity to interview Anjali Rao, an Indian American immigrant, cancer survivor, and president of the board of directors of Accessible Yoga, who offers insight into the yoga stories and histories that have been obscured by heteropatriarchy and colonization.

Anjali said, "History is being erased everywhere. History is being erased in the United States of America. It's being erased in India. It's being erased in Tibet. We are losing so many narratives, and we are left with only the dominant cultural narrative in every country."

South Asia is not a monolith. This means that even when exploring the history of yoga, there will be multiple narratives and perspectives that will depend on interpretation, inference, and the texts available versus those that have been destroyed or lost, the position and perspective of the scholar interpreting the texts, and many more factors. *That's why whom we learn from is almost as important as what we learn and how we study.*

We have to ask, whose perspective is this story written from? Who benefits from the story being written this way? Who is missing from this story?

Yoga was exported to North America from South Asia in the last hundred years or so. If a training has no connection and can't source its practices, philosophies, and techniques back to a lineage from the Indian subcontinent, then it is probably missing the heart of the practice. I see a muddling of philosophies, ideas, and New Age spirituality in many of today's teacher trainings.

I do want to say here that I have compassion and grace for (some) local yoga studios. They, too, are operating in a capitalistic world and trying to find ways to stay open. Running teacher trainings helps a lot with that. I wish more grants and venture capital funding went to local organizations and community centers run by BIPOC striving to make healing and wellness accessible to all beings.

Since teacher trainings are so expensive, this also speaks to the means of the people who can take them. And oftentimes, that is white and privileged people. I wish for more BIPOC and people who are queer or disabled to be able to take YTTs (that take their time and include history and philosophy) and create community spaces for others who can learn from them. Having spaces by BIPOC for BIPOC is crucial for the well-being of these communities.

The 200-hour YTT only scratches the surface when it comes to presenting yoga as a whole. And it is important to note that yoga also includes the reflection, integration, and application of it as well, not just cramming in the knowledge to get certified. It's a complex issue that requires a sincere rethink—and I say this as someone who teaches as a part of a 200-hour trauma-informed YTT, so I'm aware of the challenges of an imperfect system.

I wish for students, practitioners, and teachers to move toward more integrity when it comes to the preservation of yogic wisdom. This happens through continuous study, practice, and reflection. I see being a yoga teacher as a big responsibility and one that requires seriousness in practice and study. To present yoga as a whole is to understand and embody all its limbs and teachings. To share this wisdom is to be rooted in traditional teachings and texts.

Here are some solutions I think would make for better informed students and teachers. **For those that offer trainings such as yoga studios, organizations, and yoga teacher trainers, these suggestions are for you:**

We need programs, intensives, and trainings where students can study yoga and deepen their practice but *not* become a teacher at the end. Offer trainings and programs that help students go deeper into yoga rather than pushing students to become teachers. These individual programs can focus on integrating pranayama, studying the Bhagavad Gita, learning about the five Koshas and Hatha Yoga, and much more. I have found many students who want to study yoga, not teach it, but feel the only way to deepen their understanding is to attend a YTT. Let's create more in-depth study programs that are focused on helping yoga students grow and flourish.

Offer more scholarships for people who need it, particularly those who identify as BIPOC, LGBTQIA+, disabled, or who are otherwise underrepresented in the yoga and wellness space. Let's help make these trainings and programs more accessible to all people.

If you are hosting a YTT, make sure your YTT has teachers on staff who are South Asian, Black, and Indigenous, as well as other folks of color. The culture holders should not be excluded from teaching their own ancestral and spiritual practices. And only having one person of color is not enough. Let's move past tokenization as the standard. I have seen far too many homogeneous all-white teaching staffs of YTTs with a sprinkle of one person of color who is also able-bodied and of an upper class or socioeconomic background. Within the teaching staff, have a diversity of body shapes and abilities, classes, races, and genders. Students of other diverse backgrounds feel safer about joining when they see themselves represented in the teaching staff. Our identities innately affect our worldviews and beliefs. It is important to reflect that in whom you hire and learn from.

Ensure your YTT explores the depths of philosophy and history. This includes covering that yoga originated in South Asia as a pathway toward moksha and is for all beings looking to understand their mind and themselves and to reduce their suffering. Cover that yoga is over twenty-five hundred years old and how colonization, especially British colonization, impacted South Asia and yoga. Go into the depth of yogic philosophy—such as Sankhya philosophies, the Bhagavad Gita, the Yoga Sutras, and their ethical frameworks—and hire teachers who have taken the time to really know it.

Include knowledge about trans and gender-expansive identities in the training curriculum, how to build more inclusive spaces through affirming language, and make queer and trans folks feel safe and included. This can look like the use of gender-neutral terms: instead of saying "ladies and gentlemen," use terms like "everyone," "folks," or "practitioners." Hire queer and trans people to lead parts of the curriculum to offer their lived experience, knowledge, and wisdom—otherwise the YTT's continue to perpetuate cisheteronormative structures. When speaking about concepts like divine feminine and masculine energy, recognize that these traits exist in all beings, and they are not exclusive to physical sex or gender identity. Ask students for their pronouns and respect them by using the correct ones. I turn to folks in the Trans Future Collective for greater guidance here.

Teach students how to incorporate asana variations that cater to a wider range of body shapes and abilities, allowing everyone to experience the benefits of yoga. This inclusive approach fosters a stronger sense of community within the studio and opens the practice of yoga to a wider audience. The Accessible Yoga School led by Jivana Heyman does great work in this area.

Review your reading list for the training. Does it have books written by BIPOC? Are there books on the reading list that focus on decolonization and liberatory work?

These next suggestions are for yoga teachers:

I would recommend that teachers keep up their sadhana (spiritual practice) and svadhyaya (self-study and study of wisdom texts). A teacher can take a student only as far as they have gone. If a teacher has made it to just the shallow edge of the ocean, that's as far as they will be able to take their students. If a teacher has gotten to know themselves at just a surface level, it makes it much more difficult to help students know themselves deeply. Teachers should continue their own study and know this is a lifelong endeavor.

And teachers, know when to take breaks from teaching. Perhaps there will be a season or two where you go back deeper into study. Capitalism keeps us moving and hustling. Taking the time to pause and reflect is important. Teachers that teach ten to twenty yoga asana classes a week amaze me! That's a lot of space being held and energy being output. Give yourself time to rest, digest, and integrate too.

Rather than asking how you can be a better yoga teacher, I think the more worthwhile and prudent pursuit is how to be a better yoga student. It doesn't matter how many books are read and trainings are taken if the teachings remain as accumulated knowledge only. Find a teacher that resonates with you and study with them for a long time. Yes, even teachers need teachers. And know it might take some time to find a teacher you trust and with whom you resonate—be patient and, in the meantime, commit to your personal study and sadhana.

Understand that being good at asana does not equal being a good yoga teacher. Often when a student becomes proficient in asana, they are then encouraged to take the next step, which in our modern day is the teacher training. This is a huge reason why, in modern yoga, we see able-bodied or "advanced asana" practitioners as the prototype for what makes an ideal yoga teacher. However, just because you are good at teaching asana does not mean you're going to be better at teaching yoga. The only thing it means is that you are capable of and have an interest in asana, which is just one part of yoga. This excludes people who also have an interest in yoga but are not seen as the ideal teacher because of their physical ability. Being a good yoga teacher asks so much more, including: being mindful of those coming to class, caring about students, learning about philosophy, steeping yourself in tradition, and being of service. Many, if not all, of those things don't depend on physical ability or prowess.

For students who are ready and committed to being in a YTT, here are some things to look for:

1. How long has the teacher trainer been studying yoga? Do they have their own teachers they are continually studying with for ongoing guidance, growth, and inspiration?
2. Do you feel inspired and connected to the teacher as you speak with them? Do you feel that they truly see and hear you?
3. Does the teacher provide mentorship and time for one-on-one connection?
4. How long is the training? Is there enough time built in to study, reflect, and integrate?
5. Is there respect conveyed to the roots and other lineages of yoga?
6. Is the curriculum focused on yoga as a fitness modality only, or does it include history, philosophy, and the study of texts?
7. Does it seem like the training is only offered to make money? You can check if it is overpriced or if the organization pumps out training after training.
8. Is there a sliding scale, scholarships, or other financially accessible ways to take the training?

And for students contemplating taking a training, explore your intentions for doing so. If you want to go deeper into yoga or reduce stress in your life, taking a yoga series, immersion study program, or yoga course might be the better call. If you want to take it to improve your health or heal in some way, working one-on-one with a yoga teacher, yoga therapist, or Ayurvedic practitioner will be a more supportive container. There are many ways to study and go deeper into yoga beyond taking a 200-hour YTT that costs thousands of dollars.

There are yoga students and teachers who have studied under a traditional guru–shishya lineage, through a family lineage, or have done other forms of study that are not credentialed under Yoga Alliance or other Western credentialing bodies. Does this mean their knowledge and wisdom is not valid? Of course not! Indigenous and other lineage-based teachers do not need to be certified by Western standards to be validated or approved to teach.

One of my peers in the space, Abha, a lifelong yoga practitioner and neuroscientist from Nepal, shared with me that even though she grew up practicing aspects of yoga with her mom, her colleague felt that she knew more about yoga and Abha's culture after taking a YTT. Imagine the audacity. Abha shares her story:

> *Yoga is a practice that combines science and spirituality, addressing questions about the self and the purpose of existence. It seeks to provide answers through direct experience. It is fascinating to discover that the ancient Vedantic science from which yoga originated encompasses mathematical, astronomical, and medical knowledge. It's incredible to witness the resurgence of ancient yogic teachings in the West, especially considering their history of being dismissed as pseudoscience. While the West recognizes some aspects of yoga as beneficial for physical and mental well-being, it is unfortunate that in the West, the focus on yoga is often limited to its physical exercises, known as asanas. This narrow perspective overlooks the other significant dimensions of yoga contributing to its holistic nature.*
>
> *Growing up in Nepal, I practiced aspects of yoga, such as Japa, Dhyāna, and Prānāyāma, from an early age with my mother. During my post-doctoral training, I followed a [white] colleague's recommendation and started practicing yoga at a corporate studio. However, I quickly realized that*

> *this studio heavily emphasized the physical aspects of yoga, treating it more like a gymnastics workout. The primary focus was on attaining a toned physique and perfect abs. Furthermore, there was a particular emphasis on showcasing women who excelled in physically demanding poses such as handstands and chin stands. These studios also pushed me to join costly teacher training courses, capitalizing on profit. I felt uncomfortable with their tendency to exoticize and commercialize yoga's symbols, rituals, and clothing. Despite being asked frequently, I chose not to enroll in their teacher training program.*
>
> *Ironically, the colleague who recommended the studio ended up pursuing teacher training. However, she began dismissing my experiences and cultural heritage, claiming credit for my interest in yoga. She even made inappropriate comparisons between yoga and Christianity. When I raised concerns about the lack of representation for South Asians and women of color in yoga magazines, she brushed them off. Interestingly, she later married a South Indian man, which she used as a justification to diminish others' experiences. Her demeanor disheartened me, but I moved on from this experience, and it compelled me to reflect on the problematic appropriation of yoga culture.*
>
> *Everything happens for a reason, and incidents like these have motivated me to delve deeper into yoga's scientific and spiritual aspects.*

Just because this student took a 200-hour training does not mean that made her an expert on someone else's cultural heritage. Yet this type of behavior persists in the yoga space. Appropriation is rampant.

We need to bring a sense of humility and reverence back to these practices and to being a teacher.

Remember, as the teacher of yoga, you are the ultimate student in that experience. Yes, you might be guiding and leading the class, but the class of students is teaching you most of all. Every time I have led a class and held space—whether for one person, five, twenty-five, or three hundred—I walked away a little different from when I began. This is because we learn just as much as we teach and give. Remember to hold both truths.

Teachers have so much power. If we change the way we think about how yoga is taught—how students are brought in and encouraged along this path, sometimes becoming teachers themselves—then we can begin to change how our culture thinks about *yoga* itself.

11

SPIRITUAL BYPASSING WON'T SAVE US

SPIRITUAL BYPASSING is a term that has come up in spaces that I have been in quite often since 2020 in the conversation around being yoga practitioners, students, and teachers.

When my yoga colleagues and I have expressed problems we are seeing in the yoga space, I have heard people respond with the following:

- "But we are all one!"
- "But we are all consciousness!"
- "I'm sure the (Hindu) Gods and Goddesses wouldn't mind, so why do you?"
- "All lives matter."
- "I don't see color."
- "Everything is love."
- "Love and light."

These statements mean to avoid the pain of understanding, change, and true growth. This is spiritual bypassing, where spirituality is used as a shield or defense mechanism against psychological wounds, difficult emotions or experiences. It can also be used as a defense mechanism against the difficult feelings that arise when colonialism, whiteness, and cultural appropriation are confronted.

When I was living in New Orleans, I started a yoga class for people of color because I felt that it was important for folks of the global majority and those who are not often represented or seen in modern yoga classes to have a brave space to come together, build community, and practice. I say *brave* as opposed to *safe* because unfortunately we cannot guarantee safety for everyone; we do not know what trauma and triggers people are coming in with. The term "brave space" is credited to educators Brian Arao and Kristi Clemens. It emerged as a concept in their 2013 book *The Art of Effective Facilitation: Reflections from Social Justice Educators*. It was introduced as an alternative to the term "safe space" to address limitations associated with creating a completely risk-free environment for learning and dialogue. Safety cannot be guaranteed. I also felt it was important for these classes to be donation-based and financially accessible.

One day, I woke up to comments on the Facebook ad I had made from someone named Chad saying, "But isn't yoga about oneness? Why would you intentionally create more separation? This is not right."

This is a perfect example of spiritual bypassing. In falling back on language like "oneness," Chad failed to understand or confront how racially divided America is and how it was methodically created and shaped by white supremacy.

The yoga and wellness industry is a microcosm of the neocolonial reality we live in. The yoga we have inherited in the West is a product of colonial trauma, and we are causing more harm to marginalized communities when we believe light and love is the answer to the systemic oppression that centers white people as the leaders and experts of South Asian spiritual and wisdom teachings.

What Chad was also not seeing was that mainstream yoga classes are full of white people and very few people of color.

Addressing and creating solutions to something that the majority of people don't recognize as a problem perfectly demonstrates the need to draw awareness to the reality beyond the superficial understanding that pertains to an exclusive group.

The term *spiritual bypassing* was made popular in the 1980s by John Welwood, a Buddhist teacher and psychotherapist who observed the phenomenon in his own spiritual community. He defined it as "using one's spirituality to avoid facing unresolved issues either on a personal, interpersonal or systemic level."

Here are some more examples of spiritual bypassing:

Nonattachment without compassion. For instance, believing indifference equals equanimity. This might look like a person ignoring injustice or pain in the world and mistaking this attitude for spiritual peace and calm. Yes, equanimity and peace are a part of yoga and other spiritual philosophies. However, indifference to suffering is never recommended. Yoga Sutra 1.33 describes the four keys as maitri (friendship or loving-kindness toward those who are happy), karuna (compassion for those suffering), mudita (sympathetic joy to those who are virtuous), and equanimity (wise evenness of the mind toward those who are nonvirtuous). In Buddhism, these four heart and mind qualities are known as Brahmaviharas. Truly practicing these tenets, especially karuna, would mean helping someone who is suffering. Imagine a world where everyone practiced yoga in this way! As a practice, compassion opens the heart to the depth of life's beauty and pain. *Taking action to help those suffering is one of the most yogic things we can do.*

Evasion of uncomfortable feelings. Spiritual bypassing in this case includes trying to use yogic practices as a means of avoiding or suppressing emotions versus nonjudgmentally witnessing whatever arises, whether that's feelings of anger, grief, shame, jealousy, or guilt. It can also mean thinking you must "rise above" your emotions. The problem with this is that negative or unpleasant emotions are completely normal and must be felt like any other emotion. You are not a "bad" or a less enlightened being for having unpleasant feelings. When we ignore and suppress those emotions, they come out in worse ways.

Fallacious expectations. An example of such expectations is believing that practice must always be a positive experience and never challenging or uncomfortable. This can show up in the yoga teacher who tries to make sure everyone in the class is visibly having a good time or the student who only wants to go to "fun" yoga classes.

Tone policing or pacifying others. This is evident in phrases like "Shouldn't a yoga teacher be calm?", "Love and light only, please," and "Karma will figure that out." I want all yoga students, practitioners, and teachers to understand that they are allowed to have real human emotions, especially when witnessing or experiencing injustice, harm, or bypassing. We are allowed to get angry, frustrated, sad, and upset. Yoga is about discernment and justice. Our anger is valid and has tremendous power for change. Being spiritual does not mean we are cosplaying as "Zen and unattached" at all times. I find the most spiritual people are those who are deeply affected by the world around them and are doing something to make things better, not just ignoring or pretending it does not exist.

Weaponizing your spiritual practice. This form of spiritual bypassing asserts superiority over those who don't share the same practice, potentially to hide personal insecurities or as a way to avoid the internal work of investigating how a person might be complicit in systems of harm. This can also show up as someone thinking they're so "enlightened" that they can do no wrong. (News flash: even Siddhartha Gautama, the Buddha, made mistakes!)

Spiritual bypassing often creates conditions where the person sidestepping someone else's reality is thinking about only themselves while using spirituality and the practices to advance their own life. Fannie Lou Hamer's bold claim that "nobody's free until everybody's free" comes to mind here. Yoga is a path that seeks to burn away our ignorance so that we can see how interconnected we all are. My liberation is bound up in yours.

A small way we can put this into practice is by offering kindness where we can on a daily basis. Smile at the stranger you see as you walk down the street, call a friend whom you haven't spoken to for a while, donate to mutual aids and people in need. Start to see everyone as yourself.

Spiritual bypassing also ignores the dualities of life. There is joy and sadness, beauty and ugliness, pleasure and pain. Only focusing on "love and light" misses the nuances.

The real spiritual work is to see the problems and harm being caused in our physical reality and work on repairing that, not to attempt to ascend to another dimension where everything is "perfect."

Yoga in itself addresses how we are all suffering (dukkha) and provides wisdom and solutions for relief. In *Love and Rage*, Lama Rod Owens defines acceptance of reality in this context as

> *simply allowing the thing to be there, whatever the thing is. It is a practice of no judgement. . . . Accepting without judgment means we are not celebrating or denying the thing . . . We must first accept the reality of something before trying to change it. . . . This teaching can be a hard thing to hear when we are being asked to accept forms of violence or harm happening to us or others. I tell activists often that if we want to change systems of violence and inequity, we must accept the reality of these systems. Again, accepting doesn't mean celebrating or condoning; it only means that we allow the reality to be present so we can see it and really figure out how to change it. We cannot walk unless our feet are on the ground.*

The Five Kleshas

In yogic texts, the sources of suffering are *kleshas*, which translates to *poison* or *affliction*. The kleshas are considered the cause of suffering in both yogic and Buddhist philosophy and something we need to actively work to understand and overcome.

The five kleshas are as follows:

1. Avidya (ignorance): the misperception that we are limited beings and the ignorance of not knowing we are spiritual beings. This is the source of all suffering.

2. Asmita (I-am-ness): the overidentification with our ego and the false identification with self-images that we create about ourselves, which are not true: *I am a bad person*, *I am not worthy*, *I am better than that person*, or *I am never wrong*.
3. Raga (attachment): the attraction and desire for things we perceive will bring us happiness or satisfaction. This creates an endless cycle of desire–chase–receive or not-receive–suffer. Happiness is not found in the pursuit of material objects or experiences outside of ourselves.
4. Dvesha (aversion): the opposite of raga, it is the aversion and pushing away of things we think cause unpleasant sensations or experiences. It is the desire to avoid anything we dislike.
5. Abhinivesha (will to live): this is our fear of death, even though we know death is the one thing that is certain, alongside change.

To overcome the kleshas, we must first acknowledge them. This can be an uncomfortable thing to sit with, to explore our inner darkness and shadows. However, it is a crucial step in knowing ourselves and being in a better relationship with the world around us. We cannot heal, we cannot fix, and we cannot repair what we refuse to acknowledge.

Vipassana is a form of meditation that is a practical approach to *seeing reality as it is, not as we want it to be* (the literal translation of the word). In this practice, we attend to whatever arises, which includes the kleshas.

We can think of kleshas as weeds that need to be removed from the garden of our mind. To do this, we must first admit and accept that these seeds of ignorance, desire, and aversion are there in the first place—as they are for all human beings. As humans, we process our reality through our layers of conditioning, formed by society, our upbringing, samskaras, and perceptions. Each one of us has been brought up uniquely, and these intersecting identities impact our kleshas. This happens at personal, cultural, institutional, and systemic levels.

At a personal level, we all have constructed identities—or as Swami-ji referred to them, "functional identities." I identify as an able-bodied, brown, middle-class, college-educated, queer thirty-year-old American Punjabi Sikh cis woman born and raised in California. Yogic philosophy teaches that in the world of spirit, identities are meaningless. They are socially constructed and help us move through the physical world and relate to one another. Imagine I go up to someone and say, "Hi! I am a mass of atoms floating through the world; it is good to meet you." I would surely get strange looks, and people would think I had lost it!

While spiritually and in relation to myself, I can drop all functional identities, that is not true in the human, physical world. In my embodied experience, if I ignore, bypass, or deny my own or someone else's humanity, I cause harm and produce suffering. The more you understand your social advantages and disadvantages, the stronger and more mindful you become. You can use your unearned privileged to help yourself and advocate for those who may not have the same opportunities.

To have a human experience means to address the real suffering that exists here, which stems from so many things, including capitalism, racial injustice, homophobia, and transphobia.

Privilege and Responsibility

This leads to another conversation about privilege. Privilege is when certain groups of people get special benefits or easier access to things simply because of their social identity rather than because of any effort on their part. Not being able to see, recognize, or understand someone else's pain or suffering often comes from being in a place of privilege. The ability to spiritually bypass can come from a place of privilege or be a way to avoid confronting privilege.

Identities that hold privilege can include but are not limited to white privilege, white-passing privilege, cis male privilege, heterosexual privilege, cisgender privilege, socioeconomic privilege, able-bodied privilege, religious privilege, passport privilege, beauty privilege, and age privilege. In this human reality and experience, different values and meanings are associated with each identity. This shows up as the conscious or unconscious belief that *white is better than Black and brown* (racism), *male is better than female* (sexism), *young is better than old* (ageism), *able is better than disabled* (ableism), and *heterosexuality is better than homosexuality* (heteronormativity).

Cisgender and straight people often don't realize the privileges they have, like not worrying about bathroom safety or coming out. These advantages are not earned but simply exist due to their identity. I acknowledge and hold my privilege as a cis woman.

Even as a young girl, I had the sense that having lighter skin was more acceptable. Both my grandmother and mother would tell me to cover my skin when I went outside because they didn't want me to get too dark, which was seen as undesirable.

These judgments are problematic, especially when they become ingrained or normalized. As a result, discrimination becomes normalized because, of course, if that person is "less than" or "not as good as me," then (the thinking goes) I can violate their rights, exclude them, ridicule them, and at the worst of times, place their life in danger. It is avidya in action to think that someone is less than me based on their identity.

When white folks say they are color-blind, this is bypassing and racism in action. If we want humanity to have a chance, white folks need to acknowledge how every part of their lives enables white supremacy to flourish and grow. By bypassing, we are not getting to the root of racism. We aren't even trying. In *White Women: Everything You Already Know about Your Own Racism and How to Do Better*, Regina Jackson and Saira Rao write, "If all you see is white, you don't see color, right? Erasing your white power is a prerequisite to being color-blind, and color-blindness is a form of racism. If you don't see color, you don't see your white power, and if you don't see your white power, you don't see your racism. And if you don't see racism, you cannot dismantle it. If you cannot dismantle it, you are actively supporting it."

Those in positions of power have the ability to make change in this way, and everyone has the capacity to say something. We have to build and support people who challenge and disrupt systems that uphold hierarchy and inequity.

As Susanna Barkataki, yoga educator and yoga unity activist, shares, "I do think that white folks have more responsibility to look at their positionality and their privilege and to examine where they might be appropriating or taking up space or doing something to a wisdom tradition that doesn't come from their culture."

Look around your workplace, yoga studio, friend circle, and organizations. How many QTBIPOC (queer, trans, Black, Indigenous, people of color) are there? Why is that? It is the responsibility of white folks and those in power to build relationships, name sources, and invite QTBIPOC to teach and speak. For example, if you don't see a South Asian person in yoga studios, festivals, or trainings, ask why and make sure to invite and call them in. This onus cannot be placed on those with marginalized identities because marginalized folks get shunned and blacklisted for speaking up for themselves.

The Importance of Spaciousness and Mirroring

The goal of yoga, according to all traditional texts, is self-inquiry and transformation. We must acknowledge and accept the ways we cause harm to ourselves and others through our attachment to power and control, to the insidious belief that certain groups of people are better than others. This then requires taking the time to sort out harmful thought patterns and using action to purify our minds, beliefs, and actions.

This requires committing to understanding oneself and bringing compassionate inquiry and awareness to how you have been conditioned. Remaining ignorant or not going deep within doesn't make you a bad person, but the cycles of harm continue to repeat themselves into future generations.

This work is not possible without internal and external spaciousness, especially mental spaciousness. This space is always available to us if we draw our awareness to it. I have guided students in meditation to notice the space between each breath: at the top of the inhale, at the bottom of the exhale, and between each thought. To notice the space and stillness within. This space is like the container that holds all our feelings, emotions, and thoughts. We have the capacity to notice this mental spaciousness so that we can work through our triggers and biases. Think about when you are really stressed out and tense—how much spaciousness did you feel within and throughout? This constriction doesn't allow for possibilities. And conversely think about when you are relaxed and content—how much spaciousness did you feel then? When we are tense and constricted with self-righteousness or guilt, this doesn't create the space needed to objectively look at the situation and our part in it. Self-reflection and emotional awareness require mental spaciousness. This is where practices like breathing with exhales that are longer than inhales, body scan meditation, restorative yoga asana, and savasana can be incredibly useful to tune into the spaciousness that already exists and to operate from a place of connecting to the sacred pause. We don't always need to take immediate action when we are in a reactionary or triggered state.

This is where a teacher, someone you trust and have faith in, can also be supportive. Someone who truly sees you and can offer honest feedback. I can't tell you the number of times I have taken a problem to one of my teachers—questions like *How do I work with this jealousy I am experiencing? Someone said a mean thing to me, and it is really messing with me. How do I skillfully manage my reaction and emotions?* We don't need to do this alone. We can support one another on working through our insecurities and trauma.

I supported a student through her pregnancy and one of the things we worked on was her worry about unconsciously passing down ancestral curses to her child. She didn't want to recreate the cycle where she felt like her own mother wasn't emotionally available to see and hear her. We cocreated an open space and relationship where she felt brave enough to share her honest feelings and insecurity without the risk that I would judge her. We began with joint warm-ups (sukshma vyayama) to reduce physical tension, and then I had her settle into a Supported Butterfly Pose (supta baddha konasana) using bolsters, blocks, and blankets. This was to create ease for the physical body to feel grounded and settled. I then used meditation and visualization to have her bring this part of herself out and speak to it with curiosity and compassion. This part needed to be seen, heard, and loved by my student. This younger part didn't want to get further left behind when the baby was born. It wanted to be seen and loved by my student. My student realized she needed to make intentional space every day to take care of this part of herself through returning to painting (which she used to love), journaling, and sitting outside on the grass. When we really tune in, we might be surprised by the answers within and the small things we can do to take care of every part of ourselves.

The Shadow: Our Own and the Collective

We have to learn to approach our own wounds with equanimity, curiosity, and acceptance—the qualities required to heal them. Fear of the shadow, the parts of our personality that we choose to reject and repress, is understandable and deserving of compassion. Shadow work, the practice of exploring our darker aspects, has deep roots in ancient traditions across cultures, coming to us from Indigenous teachings. It is inherent to Yoga and Buddhism. While Carl Jung coined the term of *shadow self*, the concept has existed for millennia before him, often using ceremonies and rituals to explore the unconscious. Acknowledging this history highlights the universality of shadow work and its connection to ancestral wisdom, inviting us to confront and integrate our darker aspects.

The shadow self includes the aspects of ourselves that we dislike or believe society won't accept, prompting us to suppress these parts and traits deep within. Much like the way the samskaras need to be brought into the light to be healed, so do parts of our shadow. Otherwise, we are quick to point out other people's flaws or tell them how wrong they are without looking inward.

If we look at aspects of our shadow as something to learn from, this creates acceptance, and we can unlock the wisdom these parts hold. Fear can be turned into courage. Pain connects us to the fragility of the human experience and can be a catalyst for strength and resilience. Our pain can teach us that we do not want to perpetuate that to someone else, ever again, because we know how excruciating it was to experience. We can think about someone who was abused as a child, never took the time to heal from it, and then continued that same cycle of abuse with their children. On the opposite side, there are those who dove deep into their pain of childhood abuse, untangled the layers of fear, guilt, shame, sadness, and rage, learned from them, and swore to never do that to another person. I am that second person. Aggression can be transmuted into warrior-like discipline. We cannot bypass this deep inner work.

Here are some reflection questions to notice and befriend the shadow:

- What emotions do you try to avoid or deny (e.g., anger, jealousy, sadness)? What makes you afraid to feel them?
- Are there any parts of yourself you can show more compassion to (i.e., the parts of yourself you might consider lazy, judgmental, unkind, or selfish)? What medicine or wisdom does that part of you have to offer?
- Have you forgiven yourself?

- Are there any past mistakes you're still beating yourself up over?
- Is there anyone else in your life you need to forgive?
- In what ways can you care for and honor your body?
- When was the last time a person triggered you? Can you see how the aspects of that person who triggered you are also in you?

At a societal level, there also exists a collective shadow. How could there not, with thousands of years of land theft, enslavement, imperialism, colonialism, genocide, and racism? As a collective, we cannot bypass these real histories or focus only on whitewashed versions of history that seek to sanitize, rewrite, and lessen or justify oppressors' roles in such cruel and evil acts. Otherwise, these histories repeat themselves, as is currently happening at the time of writing this book with the genocide in Palestine. Whenever a group, society, or nation firmly holds its own moral righteousness, superiority, or entitlement, the collective shadow comes into play. As individuals, we must do this deep inner work, learn from marginalized communities to understand their perspectives, and commit to making the world a better place in any way that we can. As a society, we must confront this collective shadow, and we have to turn to the most oppressed peoples, elders, and Indigenous folks to guide us.

Yoga provides tools for us to skillfully understand ourselves and one another. We need spiritual spaces and yoga classes where anti-oppression is discussed, where we can use meditation to investigate and purify the mind, and where people are willing to be changed. It is time to use these tools and practices to create more humane conditions for all people to thrive and prosper, not just certain communities.

12

THE GIFT THAT YOGA GIVES US

I'M SURE MANY of us can agree that life has a baseline of struggle, angst, confusion, and anger that is just inherently a part of being alive. For some this struggle is maintained and heightened by oppressive systems like capitalism, racism, patriarchy, cisheteronormatism and other mind viruses.

We all experience life's woes. They might involve struggling to understand others—or to be understood yourself. A friend, partner, spouse, child, or boss at any point in our life could be causing us some level of grief. Perhaps you feel existential dread or fear about sickness, death, or from contemplating the state of the world.

When I close out meditation and asana practice, I always end by saying, "Thank you for the blessing of this life, the realities of all the highs and lows."

Because that is the reality of being alive as a human being—there will be highs AND there will be lows. Yoga offers us wisdom, practices, and contemplative space to find equanimity and ease through all of it.

This is one big thing in Karma yoga and what Krishna in the Bhagavad Gita teaches us: how to develop cheerfulness, contentedness, and equanimity through all of life, even in the midst of suffering.

Do I wish I could just wave a magic wand and make all my problems disappear? Sure! But unfortunately (or fortunately!), that is not the reality we live in. We have to learn how to move with grace (and sometimes big ol' adult tantrums) through life.

So much of the yogic path is learning how to deal with human struggle with more equanimity and grace.

One of the main problems yoga points to is that our wants (ragas) and dislikes (dveshas) are unlimited. This causes problems because we are always searching, clamoring, and wanting more of what we think is desirable and pushing away what we think is undesirable.

Oftentimes, it is as if we are looking to the future where everything will be better—once we have that new job, are making more money, have a perfect partner, have a "better" body—and only then will real happiness be found. I want to encourage us to take a deep breath right here and say, "This is the main show. I am living my life right now."

Happiness and joy are innately within us.

***

This attempt to address human suffering has actually been present in yoga from the very beginning in the core concepts of samsara and moksha.

Samsara refers to the cycle of birth–death–rebirth, an endless cycle characterized in part by suffering. Samsara is characterized by suffering and dissatisfaction. It is viewed as a cycle of endless desires (raga), aversions (dvesha), attachments, and ego-driven actions that perpetuate the cycle of rebirth (as outlined in the previous chapter's section on kleshas). The ultimate goal in many dharmic traditions, including yoga, is to break free from the cycle of samsara and attain liberation or enlightenment, known as moksha (in Hinduism and Sikhism) or nirvana (in Buddhism and Jainism). By having a cessation of craving and attachment and living ethically, seekers can break free from this cycle of samsara. Moksha can also be understood as self-realization and enlightenment in *this* lifetime.

In the Yoga Sutras, samadhi is understood as the highest state of consciousness in yoga, representing the state of union with the divine or ultimate reality. It is a state of profound absorption, where the practitioner transcends the limitations of the ego and experiences pure consciousness and bliss. In yoga, moksha is a present-moment experience. It is seen as the realization of one's true nature and the recognition that the individual self is interconnected with the universal consciousness.

Moksha can be achieved by becoming more enlightened and more self-realized than you were in the days, weeks, months, years, or even lifetimes before. It's like the peeling of an onion—we are always learning more about ourselves.

Moksha is a state of profound self-realization, where the individual transcends the limitations of the ego and experiences their true nature, which is believed to be eternal, blissful, and interconnected with the ultimate reality. Dr. Neil Dalal, a professor of South Asian philosophy and religious thought, said to me, "All of the classical yoga traditions were pursuing moksha. If moksha gets taken out, is it still yoga?"

I believe this is an excellent question. **Without some attempt to alleviate human suffering on a psychological, spiritual, and collective level, modern yoga may not be truly yoga.**

Human or Robot?

In Becky Chambers's novel *A Psalm for the Wild-Built* (which I highly recommend), there is a scene where Sibling Dex, a traveling tea monk, is having a conversation with a robot who has been freed from forced labor. This is set in a future where artificial intelligence and machines have become sentient enough to want to revolt from being forced to work for humans.

Sibling Dex admits to feeling unfulfilled even though he serves tea to different villages, listens to people's problems, and makes a positive impact. But he still feels like something is missing. He feels like *he needs a purpose to truly live*—like he needs to make something of his life.

At one point, Sibling Dex says, "I don't know. I don't know what is wrong with me. Why isn't it enough? What am I supposed to do, if not this? What *am* I, if not this?"

How many of us can relate to this feeling? Even though I have a committed partner, even though I have work that fulfills me where I know I am making a difference, even though I have friends who love me, still at times I feel this yearning for something more. At times, even with a full schedule, my anxiety keeps pushing me to strive to achieve more, to attain more. *More, more, more.*

In *A Psalm for the Wild-Built,* the robot responds to Sibling Dex by saying that he thought humans, as an advanced species, understood their place. Sibling Dex protests that they do understand their place. But the robot disagrees:

> *You're an animal, Sibling Dex. You are not* separate *or* other. *You're an animal. And animals have* no purpose. *Nothing has a purpose. The world simply* is. *If you want to do things that are meaningful to others, fine! Good! So do I! But if I wanted to crawl into a cave and watch stalagmites with Frostfrog for the remainder of my days, that would also be both fine and good. You keep asking why your work is not* enough, *and I don't know how to answer that, because it is enough to exist in the world and marvel at it. You don't need to justify that, or earn it. You are allowed to just* live. *That is all most animals do.*

Sibling Dex replies that he simply wants something more. And the robot's next response is something I haven't been able to stop thinking about:

> *And I'm saying that I think you are mistaking something learned for something instinctual.*

This is at the crux of why so many of us feel unhappy. It is how the machine of colonialism and capitalism keeps us churning. We have been taught to associate our value with our productivity. We are only as worthy as the size of our bank account, the number of social media followers we have, how productive we are for our employers, the size of our house. Capitalism is intentionally designed to keep people stressed and financially insecure. This constant state of worry makes workers easier to exploit, with lower wages and poorer working conditions. When people are focused on survival, they have less time and energy to challenge the system itself.

My generation was put on a hamster wheel at a young age—chasing good grades for gold stars to be moved onto the next level, to do well at our extracurriculars for college applications, to attend great colleges, to get good jobs, to pay our bills, to purchase cars, to buy houses . . . and to pay for therapy to help us feel better when all of the aforementioned fails to satisfy us.

At some point, while working at a job I was good at, I was still exhausted and unhappy and left with the question, Is this all there is to life? This was when yoga—true yoga—came to me. Yoga came with the answers and self-inquiry tools to make sense of this life we are given.

Yoga, like the robot speaking to Sibling Dex, made me see that there is nothing wrong in having wants and ambitions. But if I were to fulfill none of them, that would be okay. We are allowed to be happy simply because we exist and are alive.

I'm going to say that again because it's so important. *We are allowed to be happy simply because we exist and are alive.*

At a ten-day silent Vipassana meditation retreat in Queensland, Australia, I had a profound realization.

When it came to my turn to meet with the assistant teacher, an Australian woman with short gray hair in a beige outfit, seated in Sukhasana and gazing down at me from her slightly elevated seat, I asked, "Okay, so what the teachings are saying is that it is okay to pursue goals and plan for the future, *but* when that pursuit starts to make us miserable, we should *just give up that goal*?"

She smiled down at me. "Exactly. Your peace of mind is important. If this pursuit is making you this miserable, then maybe it's time to let it go."

I pondered this. Most of my life I had been taught that quitting and giving up on something was a sign of failure—that somehow I had not succeeded or lived up to my potential. And here, meditating six to eight hours per day, I was learning that perhaps it was time to unlearn some, if not most, of what I had been taught and conditioned to believe.

Yoga is really a process of learning and unlearning. And then learning and unlearning some more. To drop the conditioning we have picked up over time that makes us miserable, that makes us not see ourselves as whole, that makes us discontent.

I tried to verbalize my realization with the assistant teacher. "Is it because I have an attachment to the end result, needing it to look or turn out a certain way?" I asked. "That attachment is causing me suffering. So it is also important to enjoy the present moment instead of being so focused on the outcome and thinking that happiness will only be reached when I hit my goal. Because that outcome could turn out to be different than what I imagine anyways."

She nodded, pleased. "Exactly."

As the cliché goes, tomorrow is not promised, and what we have is today. Getting too obsessed and attached to a future outcome and needing it to turn out a certain way is a recipe for suffering. We can control only what we can control. The rest, we must let go.

One of the most quoted verses of the Bhagavad Gita reminds us of this as well: "You have a right to perform your prescribed duties, but you are not entitled to the fruits of your actions. Never consider yourself to be the cause of the results of your activities, nor be attached to inaction" (2.47).

Do your work to the best of your ability, with your current conditions, and don't get attached to the outcome and the results. An affirmation I will mentally repeat to myself when perfectionism rears its head is, *I am doing the best I can with what I have in this moment and that is enough.*

Verse 2.48 provides us with another definition of yoga: "Remaining steadfast in yoga, oh! Dhananjaya, perform actions, abandoning attachment, remaining the same to success and failure alive. This evenness of mind is called yoga."

This evenness of mind is called yoga. It is to accept success and failure, pleasure and pain, as a part of life and to learn to embrace both equally. We learn to see every experience of life as a gift to practice equanimity and refine our mind.

The Gift or Curse of Self-Awareness

One big lesson yoga philosophy taught me is radical self-love, to become my own biggest fan and to have my own back—no matter what happens. An affirmation that has been helpful for me is *No matter what happens, Harpinder, I will never abandon you.*

Many of us let fear of failure hold us back from pursuing our dreams. This can lead to regret and a strained relationship with oneself. Perhaps the greatest fear is confirming our own doubts. But what if failure wasn't the end, but a stepping stone? Embracing the possibility of falling short while still valuing ourselves is crucial to personal growth and fulfillment. What would it look like to say that even if *I fail at this, I will still love and celebrate myself, because I know I gave it an honest try*?

In *A Psalm for the Wild-Built*, Sibling Dex at one point asks the robot, "It doesn't bother you? The thought that your life might mean nothing in the end?"

The robot responds,

> *That's true for all life, I've observed. Why would it bother me? Do you not find consciousness alone to be the most exhilarating thing? Here we are, in this incomprehensibly large universe, on this one tiny moon around this incidental planet, and in all the time this entire scenario has existed, every component has been recycled over and over and over again into infinitely incredible configurations, and sometimes, those configurations are special enough to be able to see the world around them. You and I—we're just*

> atoms *that arranged themselves the right way, and we can* understand *that about ourselves. Is that not amazing?*

How can we tap into this sense of awe that somehow we are alive in this moment? That I am writing these words on my laptop, seated at my desk, and that someday, you, my beloved friend, will be reading this book? How many circumstances had to come into play to make this possible?

For ancient yogis, breathing was more than just a biological function or personal experience. It wasn't just about the air going in and out of the body. Instead, they saw it as a spiritual practice that connected them to something much larger—the universe on a cosmic level. To breathe is to be in communion with the world around us—it is a bridge between the self and the infinite. The air we breathe has been around for billions of years—it is the same air breathed by dinosaurs millions of years ago. The food we consume, the water we drink, is all made of molecules that have been circulating around since the beginning of time. When we take part in life, we are connecting to all those that existed before us. All beings. *How wondrous is that?*

This eternal circulating life energy and life force is known as *prana*, which is in all living things. Remember how interconnected we all are!

When I was studying at an ashram in Mysore, Swamiji Prabodh Chaitanya, the philosophy teacher and Yoga-Vedanta scholar shared two things that set us apart from other species and are the two advantages of being reborn into a human body: the fact that we are *self-aware* and have *free will.*

I scribbled those notes down in my journal and then looked up at him as he continued with a depth of profoundness in his voice:

"That can be a gift or a curse depending upon you."

That was an ultimate mic drop moment for me.

To be self-aware is to have the ability to perceive and understand the things that make you who you are as an individual, including your personality, actions, values, beliefs, emotions, and thoughts. It is being able to recognize that you are alive in this body, in this time–space continuum. Self-awareness is also our ability to recognize our own experiences as living beings interacting with the world around us. We can use self-awareness to drop in, tune in, and recognize where we have room for growth, where we can grow our capacity for compassion and empathy, and where we might be causing harm—either to ourselves or to other beings.

This self-awareness is a gift when we recognize *I am not bound to my conditions or limitations. I can change my beliefs and thoughts. Every day is a new day.*

Since we are self-aware, yoga asks us to ask and figure out *Who am I?*

We are currently the only known species that is aware of its own mortality and death. Death is one of the few things that is absolutely certain. One day, I will pass away, and so will everyone that I love.

Having that knowledge can feel like a curse at times. It's why I sometimes feel this sense of learned urgency to make the most of my limited lifetime.

Yoga has given me this lesson: that no matter what I achieve or do not achieve, I am still wonderful and divine just as I am. That it is a gift to simply be alive. Yoga teaches us that we are already whole and complete. There is nothing that needs to be done or accomplished or said to prove that—now isn't that the ultimate freedom and liberation? What if we truly believed that? How would our world change?

This is drastically different from the way yoga is sold to us now—as another vehicle for merciless self-improvement. As a practice that requires us to look a certain way (thin, able-bodied), have certain things (the newest yoga mat and matching spandex set), and visit a certain location (the trendy studio). This yoga teaches us we need yoga and other things to be whole when yogic philosophy teaches us we are *already* whole. We don't need any of that. This is the lie of rampant commodification: that we need certain things to be whole.

True yoga teaches the opposite of the messaging I have received my entire life. I was taught conditional love in the relationships that I have to myself and with others. I was taught by my parents that I was lovable only if I became a doctor or lawyer. I was taught by Western beauty standards that I was lovable only if I had blond hair and blue eyes. I was taught I was lovable only if I accomplished great things in my life.

I want us all to drop these expectations of ourselves. We are lovable simply because we exist.

No matter what, you are wonderful. You belong.

I want us to go after great things that light us up—and if we choose to rest or give up, to celebrate that choice as well. May we rest our weary bones and know, still, that we will be supported by the universe and the divine.

To have free will is to have the ability to make choices that are not determined by outside factors or forces. It is the power of self-determination, the ability to choose one's own course of action. It is the choice that I get to make when I wake up in the morning and decide whether to do my sadhana (spiritual practice) or watch the news.

I know when I take that thirty to ninety minutes every morning to begin my day by meditating, practicing Nadi Shodhana and Bhramari Pranayama, praying at my altar, standing outside under the sunshine, moving my body through asana, and reading a wisdom text—through all of this—I am donning a shield of armor that will serve to protect me and bring me ease from the realities of daily life, where receiving or seeing unexpected news can be nervous-system rattling. It is the personal choice I got to make when I decided to listen to that voice of wisdom that told me to stop drinking alcohol, that it was poisoning me.

We can make the choice to learn more about yoga, about ourselves, and become more mindful beings.

This is the gift that yoga gives us.

13

RECLAIMING ANCESTRAL CONNECTION ONE STEP AT A TIME

TO THOSE OF us who have faced colonization, assimilation, forced migration, or immigration or who are children and descendants of people who faced colonization, this is for you. I understand from an embodied place what it feels like to lose touch with my cultural, ancestral, and spiritual practices. To wonder, *Where do I belong?* And then to see my ancestral practices being sold back to me, stripped of context and wisdom. I want to remind us that this inherent wisdom is within us—it is not something that can ever be taken away. All we have to do is make an intention to reclaim it, to honor our ancestral practices, and to rebuild a connection.

A few years ago, I received a message loud and clear that it is important, if not absolutely imperative, to connect to our roots and ancestors. This is a message that was recurring through my practices. In one guided meditation by an Indigenous shamanic practitioner, with the help of my animal guide, I traveled through the beautiful gloomy forest to meet with my spirit guides—my healed ancestors. (As a necessary aside, I think it is important to learn certain practices and traditions and to be guided by people who have been steeped in that culture and heritage and come from that ancestry. This is one huge reason it was important for me to find an Indigenous shamanic practitioner to lead me through this journey. This is serious work that is being done, and I don't take it lightly.)

I was guided through a forest of tall, lush trees to a blue, sparkling lake, where I saw my bibiji (grandma), someone who looked vaguely like my nanaji (grandpa), and two other figures I couldn't make out. The whole time they spoke in Punjabi with me, and I felt in my body the love and support that I have from them. My ancestors spoke of the importance of learning my Punjabi roots, becoming fluent in my native tongue, becoming more connected to Sikhism, and the importance of this connection. I was reminded to continue on this spiritual path and to keep coming back to them through this shamanic sound journey, yoga asana, meditation, pranayama, prayer, and faith. I was told by my ancestors to know this wisdom lives within my bones and DNA. They spoke to me about the importance of social justice and of being a part of positive change—that it is my duty to end generational traumas.

They also reminded me that they are always there for me and love me with such ferocity. That ancestors are always there for us. We just have to make an intention to build a relationship with them.

After this, I placed a picture of my bibiji on my altar. Every morning when I meditate and pray, I continue that relationship with her. I can ask her for guidance and support. My bibiji, when earthside, was a strong, fiery woman who raised eight children and was outspoken in pointing out right from wrong. She was there for my family during a time of intense trauma and confusion when I was only ten years old. I had blocked out this part of my life for so long that my mom had to remind me that I shared a small room with my grandmother during this time. And now she is always here for me. I get a little teary-eyed feeling her love for me. We all have healed ancestors who care this deeply for us.

As Ehime Ora, African scholar and priestess, shared in an Instagram post, "Your ancestors extend all the way back to the beginning of time and stardust. The ancestral lineage is a direct bridge and connecting piece to the Creator and source. When we acknowledge them, we acknowledge the presence of holy divinity in our own lives." Ash Johns, an ancestral healer and spiritual life coach, talks about the importance of calling on *healed* ancestors—those who want the best for us and can support us. Not all ancestors are well, are healed, have our best interests in their heart, or have the capacity to support us.

I encourage you to sit in meditation and see who shows up for you. Pray and ask for help and guidance from your healed ancestors. One of my teachers, Aja, the spirit guide coach, shared with me that you don't need to have met or known this ancestor in person. This can be a huge relief for those of my kin who have been adopted or in other ways feel a disconnect from their ancestors or family of origin. Trust who shows up and be patient. You can also ask your parents, aunts, uncles, and grandparents about your lineage.

I have found great healing in joining communities for women of color, going back to the gurdwara to pray as an adult, and learning yoga from South Asian teachers. There is power in having a base level of understanding and kinship with others who understand how I grew up because they grew up in a similar way. (I also want to prioritize finding and creating spaces where folks are talking about things like dismantling comparison, internalized oppression, et cetera; otherwise, we end up recreating cycles of harm even in BIPOC spaces.)

Part of my life's journey has been to reclaim my heritage and my culture and to recenter myself in my own life. Colonization aimed to disconnect us (BIPOC, folks of the global majority, and LGBTQIA+ people) from Spirit, our intuition, the earth, ancestral wisdom, and practices. However, when we live in combination with Spirit, we are more fully aware of our life—of our power and our intuition. A sense of wholeness returns.

Traditional teachings remind me that yoga is not only a practice but also a way of being. Every moment when we are aware, we are in the state of yoga. Each moment, each interaction, each person we come in contact with, and each experience we have is an opportunity to be in right conduct and to operate out of complete awareness. It allows us to be transformed by life.

As Sister Dang Nghiem shared in her book *Flowers in the Dark*, "Our spiritual life gives us a second chance. In fact, we have a new opportunity every time we are mindful of what is arising in us and around us. This is also the practice of being our own soul mate—remembering, knowing, and taking care of ourselves."

This reminds me that *our life is the practice*. Everything is interrelated and interconnected. We can always begin anew. To be spiritual is to commit to a way of thinking and behaving that honors this truth of interconnectedness.

There are four areas where I think we need to have a connection to be truly well. Thank you to Native American tribes and Indigenous traditions for reframing the way I think on this.

1. Spirituality (Creator, God/Goddess, the Divine, Mother Earth, Ancestors, and Spirit Guides)

What higher power do you believe in and anchor into? Who do you acknowledge and celebrate? This is where yogic ideas of faith (sraddha) and surrender to a higher power (ishvara pranidhana) come into play in our lives. Faith in something greater than ourselves and surrendering to the knowledge we are not in complete control of our life.

I love the way bell hooks describes spirituality in her book *All About Love*:

> *When I speak of the spiritual, I refer to the recognition within everyone that there is a place of mystery in our lives where forces that are beyond human desire or will alter circumstances and/or guide and direct us. I call these forces 'divine spirit.' When we choose to lead a spirit-filled life, we recognize and celebrate the presence of transcendent spirits. Some people call this presence soul, God, the Beloved, higher consciousness, or higher power. Still others say that this force is what it is because it cannot be named. To them it is simply the spirit moving in and through us.*

In Vedic philosophy, we can turn to this all-pervading and formless God as the creator of all and the creation itself. This as an embodied teaching is to see everything as sacred and worthy of worship. Your body, another person, a squirrel, a tree, the air you breathe, the cup you drink from—all sacred and worthy of worship.

When I was in India on a taxi ride from the airport to the Sivananda Ashram in Kerala, we pulled over to repair a hole in the car's tire. After getting out of the car, I stretched my legs and looked around. We were at an intersection surrounded by people on foot, in buses, on motorcycles, in cars and taxis. A few stray dogs walked by, not paying any attention to me. Immediately to the right of the tire repair shop was a small temple with a picture of Goddess Bhadrakali. Around the stone were marigold flowers, and in front of the picture were incense and other offerings people had left, like dry foods, candles, and flower petals. This felt in opposition but also fitting to the environment, where there was trash all over the dirt road. This was not a sterile, controlled environment in any way. One of my friends and colleagues in the space, Mx. Puja Singh, has shared that they feel the presence of God in everything in India. Even in this busy intersection, next to a small, worn-down tire shop, there is a small temple where people can pay their respects and leave offerings.

We do not need to go to a certain place to worship (although it can help). We can connect to spirit here and now. We can operate with an understanding that there are forces much more powerful and in control than us. We can surrender, ask for support, and be divinely guided. We can sink our hands into the soil, bury offerings to a tree of choice, and let the earth be there for us. We can turn to Mother Earth for her guidance and strength, to hold us.

Spirit lives within all creation and beyond. Yoga brought me this embodied and realized understanding, and it brought me to my knees. I am a spiritual being and get to live my life with this truth. I get to commit to a life of compassion, justice, love, and service.

2. Community (Family and Chosen Family, Your Support System, Heart Friends, and Sangha)

We need people in our lives who can see and hear us and love and support us. Who understand us. We need folks who can lovingly guide us back when we make mistakes or cause harm, those who can hold us with accountability.

Community is vital for our well-being as humans—we need one another. We need to build and have strong, loving support systems and communities, not for *if* we fail but for *when* we fail. It's inevitable that we are going to fall down and need help. To think otherwise is to reject the humanness of us all.

This makes me think of the concept of karuna (one of the Brahmaviharas and from Yoga Sutra 1.33) and having compassion. Karuna, or compassion, means understanding that we are all bound to the same vulnerability of being human. We are all going to have loss, go through unexpected changes, and die. A part of our work, then, is to cultivate compassion for ourselves and one another, to create and sustain loving communities of interdependence, trust, and love.

I spent a lot of time from my teens to my late twenties convinced that I was unlovable and unsupported and that I would end up unhoused someday (beliefs brought on and reaffirmed through life's struggles). When I left for college, my parents made it clear they would not support me because they did not want me to leave their house as an unmarried woman. I felt untethered, without a safety net to fall back on if I made a mistake. Meeting my partner, Ali, and becoming his family transformed what community means for me. I saw how supported he is by his family, their unconditional love, something I had never seen before, only read about in novels. Even then, it took three years of continuous work with my therapist to feel that I could trust my partner and be supported by him.

How many of us feel this way? One mistake away from everything being taken away from us? The way our society is structured is unforgiving. May we build resilient and loving webs of support and nourish the relationships that we have around us.

I owe so much to my spiritual teachers and the sanghas that I have been a part of, where I have received understanding and wisdom. We can turn to spiritual communities and the people within them in times of need, when we require advice, safety, or strength. While no one else can walk on the path of yoga for us, we can still be supported by sangha to keep us anchored and supported. Sangha reminds us that we are not only responsible for our own growth but for creating conditions that foster an environment of well-being and growth for others.

I give thanks to the communities and sanghas that I have been a part of over the last ten-plus years: Deer Park Monastery, Living Now Yoga, Tejal Yoga, Vipassana meditation group, Wholistic Community, Spirit Rock, Dr. Neil Dalal's Bhagavad Gita study group, Cosmic Labyrinth collective, and more.

Community is also necessary to provide a mirror for us and to make sure we remain in integrity. Group members can hold one another accountable for living up to shared values and provide guidance and wisdom on navigating ethical dilemmas. Humans are not perfect and by fostering an environment of understanding and support, a spiritual community can help individuals learn from their mistakes and emerge stronger. Open communication and a commitment to collective learning are essential for maintaining integrity within a group.

3. Environment (Daily Life, Nature, and Balance)

Humans are inherently connected to the natural world. Indigenous wisdom teaches us that we are part of, not apart from, our environment. There is no superior or inferior being or thing; all exist in interconnected harmony. Prana, this energetic life force and life-sustaining energy, flows through everything, animating everything living, nonliving, visible, and nonvisible. As Indu Arora says in her book *Yoga:*

Ancient Heritage, Tomorrow's Vision, "Prana is the cosmic current, the cosmic pulsation, the cosmic rhythm, and the cosmic movement."

Every morning, I stand outside in the sun and feel the warmth on my face. The sun is the ultimate source of prana. A part of my santosha (contentment practice) has been to offer gratitude to the sun daily. Without it, nothing would be alive.

Our tree and plant allies supply us with oxygen while we produce carbon dioxide for them. This beautiful exchange keeps all of life going. We've become separated from nature, from trees, and from animals. There have been many points in my life when I have gone out into the forest, surrounded by trees that are hundreds of years old (and even thousands of years old!), with a question, needing support, and the answers arrived. I have asked for guidance from the trees and received wisdom.

A part of this practice can be to express gratitude before you eat for the food you have and all the conditions that made it possible for you to be able to eat. The nuns I met at Deer Park Monastery were an example for this. Before eating, we would all pause, close our eyes, offer gratitude, and once the bell rang, we then ate. This pause brought more intention and meaning into the food—we consumed not just food, but food infused with gratitude.

I encourage all of us to live in accordance with and in harmony with nature. Just as the seasons change, plants bear fruit and die, days get darker and colder, and birds migrate, we change and fluctuate. It is not possible to be in bloom or to harvest success all year round. Nature teaches us this. We, too, must hibernate, go within, introspect, and take time to rest. My cat Alfy is one of my teachers. I notice how her sleeping patterns, play time, and routine intuitively change with the seasons. As soon as the season transitions to fall, she begins sleeping more and shifts where she sleeps.

As Tricia Hersey reminds us in her powerful book *Rest Is Resistance: A Manifesto*, "Our drive and obsession to always be in a state of 'productivity' leads us to the path of exhaustion, guilt, and shame. We falsely believe we are not doing enough and that we must always be guiding our lives toward more labor. The distinction that must be repeated as many times as necessary is this: We are not resting to be productive. We are resting simply because it is our divine right to do so."

Take a look at your life. How often are you in communion with the rivers, the ocean, the trees, the animals, and the soil? We find healing by being intertwined with nature, not separated and isolated from it. I sense the immense grief and loss here, that we live in such separated ways now. It was never meant to be like this, where we can go days, weeks, months, even lifetimes disconnected from nature's profound beauty and the wild.

In Francis Weller's *The Wild Edge of Sorrow*, he points to this grief as a forgetting of our inherent belonging to the world around us: "We forget we are all tangled together in this nest of life, that the air we breathe is shared, as is our water and soil, and everything is bound together in a seamless web of life. When we forget, we are able to do untold damage to our watersheds, to one another, and to the entire earth."

We need to rebuild these connections and have rituals to hold space for our sorrow over these unimaginable losses that continue to happen. We aren't meant to be happy all the time. With such loss happening around us all the time, how could that even be possible? We need ritual in connection with nature and to be in communion with one another. To be able to hold the world's and our own grief. Naomi Shihab Nye, a contemporary Palestinian American poet, says it so beautifully in her poem "Kindness":

> *Before you know kindness as the deepest thing inside,*
> *you must know sorrow as the other deepest thing.*
> *You must wake up with sorrow.*
> *You must speak to it till your voice*
> *catches the thread of all sorrows*
> *and you see the size of the cloth.*

May we connect to our sorrow and grief to tend to it, to tend to the earth and nature around us. To connect to our humanity.

4. Self (Inner World of Passions, Your Thoughts and Patterning, Your Values)

We have an entire world within us. There is a reason for the adage "All of the answers already lie within you." When I work with my students, sometimes I will share that the most important relationship they will have in this lifetime is the one they have with themselves. We need wisdom, tools, and elders to guide us in how to build this connection with ourselves and the space and quiet to deeply listen within.

When I think about the relationship we have with ourselves, I think, *Are you living a life in alignment with your passions, values, and ethics? Have you taken the time to discover what these are for you?* Otherwise, we become instilled with the values and dogma of society and others.

Ayurveda, meaning *the science of life* in Sanskrit and known as the complementary path to yoga, reminds us of the wholeness of our human experience. What we consume (food, drinks, media, sensory input), how we sleep and when we wake up, our thinking patterns, lifestyle, and our nature are considered. There must be harmony in our energy. Turning back to this thousands-year-old healing science transformed my life.

This work is about deprogramming and having a relationship with our ancestors and nature. All the wisdom and knowledge we could ever seek is already within our bones. It was never lost, only obscured by layers of violence.

It is important for us as the global majority to connect with our ancestral and spiritual practices, culture, and heritage. This can look like connection through eating food and learning recipes, through connecting to herbs, learning and practicing rituals, and learning the language, history, and the Indigenous healing practices such as yoga, Reiki, traditional Chinese medicine, Hoodoo, Brujería, and more. Find a way to connect with your motherland. That rooting and reconnection is important and healing.

I want to encourage us to dance and sing. Our bodies hold so much wisdom. Thich Nhat Hanh says, "If you look deeply into the palm of your hand, you will see your parents and all generations of your ancestors. All of them are alive in this moment. Each is present in your body. You are the continuation of each of these people." We are walking embodiments of our ancestors. We must learn to express the depths from within through dance, song, and chant—as a way for them to be realized in this physical dimension. This is one way we find freedom, when we break the chains that keep us small, unexpressed, and meek to express ourselves without apology. So what if you dance or sing badly? Is a song kept within that is bursting to come out not a worse pain? My ancestors knew the power and healing in coming together to sing and dance in times of celebration, in worship, and in times of great pain and grief.

I have found some of the greatest freedom on a dance floor, dancing ecstatically with my friends, as much as I have seated in a gurdwara singing Shabads, songs of devotion, together as a sanghat. **Liberation is not found through only one vehicle or medium.** There are many pathways and keys to the same door.

As the descendants, we are here to heal the generational cycles (both seven generations back and generations years forward) and continue the legacy of our culture and traditions. We carry both trauma and resilience.

This is something we discussed in depth during the Womxn of Color Summit, an organization I helped cofound and ran for three years, which celebrates women of color who embody their truest creative and authentic potential to make impactful change. We reflected on how to reclaim and reconnect with our ancestral practices. We also touched on the grief that comes up in realizing how much has been lost, stolen, appropriated, and forgotten in assimilation, colonization, and other genocides and moves. We knew that healing occurred when stories were shared in brave spaces.

This community was really created out of these questions: Why were we still seeing white experts and white participants centered in the healing and wellness spaces? Why were we continuing to reward colonizers taking from and profiting from technologies and wisdom traditions from Indigenous people around the world with our time and energy?

I knew there was something wrong with this spiritual erasure when the names of inspiring Black, Indigenous, and women of color (BIWOC) teachers, healers, guides, mediums, coaches, and leaders were not celebrated, amplified, or even known at all. I knew creating community was important for us to heal together. To speak on these truths, to share our grievances without needing to overexplain ourselves, and to be held with love.

One of my students and friends, Aqsa M, a South Asian Muslim and lifelong practitioner, shared her story of reclaiming for this book:

> *Western yoga is a dilution. A hint of smoke without the actual heat of flame. That echo from three caverns down. A thread of mountain wind felt at sea level. But once you step forward—feel a touch of yoga's millennia—you realize that Western yoga is mere shadow work of the real.*
>
> *Western yoga exists on a spectrum of harm and—at its extreme—is antithetical to yoga. I find it hard to enter such spaces, and when I do, very often I am angry. My body emits rage. Those around me sense it. Their gaze rests momentarily on my simmering form before shifting away. My anger is a guardian against the injustice around me: harm that comes from exclusivity and erasure. There is the advertised body, producing shame. I'm not flexible enough—I can't move like that. As if only the able-bodied can access yoga. The microaggression in terminology. Imperialism is present here*

when the Western practitioner fails to acknowledge the source of their knowledge. The original teachers resided an ocean away, dark-skinned and who you called archaic. Yet here is your descendant selling me ancient knowledge of the brown and Black bodies dressed in "civilized" clothing. There is violence in such spaces, when the teacher claims the blue-sky day so beautiful without naming the nation of those who held the earth in such care before the colonizer's exploitation. I practice on the unceded land of the Muskogee, also known as Atlanta, Georgia.

Western yoga isolates the individual from their creation community. It halts at the bodily sense of self and stops short of the unity at the core of yoga. When was the last time I entered a Western practice space and asked to rebuild my relationship with the earth that I harmed? How often are we encouraged by our teachers to engage in social justice movements, to understand that systematic inequities keep us from the spiritual yoke?

My practice is a decolonization of this harm and a life lived more consciously toward the divine. A return to the lessons already in my skin. This is my ancestral narrative. To formulate a conduct of living with lesser harm—ahimsa—*and a path toward truth*—satya. *It is a means for me, and I am a means for an inching truth of its name.*

Reclaiming means giving room for the anger to be alive. To honor the parts of us that say, hey this is not right. Our anger is sacred and comes with a message that needs to be heard.

Amelia Butler, an Indigenous Māori woman of Ngātiwai, Ngāti Awa, and Ngāpuhi descent and director of Learn Māori Abroad, speaks of the term *reindigenization*. Reindigenization is "about reclaiming, reconnecting, and remembering our indigenous culture." It decenters the colonizer and brings the focus back to the Indigenous person. Many of us are not Indigenous and, in fact, are uninvited settlers on Indigenous lands (or those whose ancestors were forcibly brought over), yet this serves as a reminder for all of us to reconnect to our own cultures, whatever they might be. It is a process of unlearning and remembering.

With every action we take, we are constantly asking ourselves the same questions we are asking of the world: How can we be aware of when we are still using the master's tools to create a new and more just world, and how can we imagine something better?

Audre Lorde says,

> *For the master's tools will never dismantle the master's house. They may allow us to temporarily beat him at his own game, but they will never enable us to bring about genuine change. Racism and homophobia are real conditions of all our lives in this place and time. I urge each one of us here to reach down into that deep place of knowledge inside herself and touch that terror and loathing of any difference that lives here. See whose face it wears. Then the personal as the political can begin to illuminate all our choices.*

Our commitment to wellness is about saying *yes* to a journey of starting and staying on the path of collective liberation. It is not only about self-care as bubble baths but instead about genuine change. When we reconnect to our spirituality, this provides greater healing, understanding, and liberation. These traditions have been suppressed and demonized for centuries by European slave owners, colonialists, and neocolonialists all over the world.

In many countries—like Cuba, Brazil, Haiti, and Trinidad—European colonists and slave masters attempted to obliterate the humanity and autonomy of enslaved Africans. They were often forbidden from practicing their Indigenous religions and other religions like Islam.

Christianity was marked as the only proper religion, and people were forced to give up their religions. Stigma against dharmic religions like Hinduism and Sikhism, as well as African spirituality and paganism, still exists. The Roman Catholic Church has often viewed these practices as akin to demon worship, and I have spoken to many practitioners of yoga who shared how their parents thought they were doing devil worship and were worshipping statues. I have seen TikTok videos of (misinformed) people, mostly Christians, talking about how yoga is demonic. What greatly troubles me here is the closed-mindedness. I am a huge proponent for interfaith understanding and worship. Over history, Christian missionaries have made it their mission to convert people. This has caused great violence, demonized people, and disconnected them from their own faith. This is something we all need to heal from. There is a past that has not been reconciled and needs to be worked through. As Dr. Jenn M. Jackson shared, "Whenever Black and Brown people resist oppression, we are cast as violent, aggressive, and riotous. But the oppressors are silent about the violence they've enacted, typically for generations. This is how colonization works. Rewriting history is central to this process."

Our understanding and grasp of our cultures, traditions, and practices is impacted by us having lost our ancestral heritage by being uprooted from our motherlands or born as first- or second-generation immigrants in Western countries. I have felt caught between worlds, not really Indian enough but also not American enough. Many of us might feel guilt, shame, confusion, anger, frustration, and grief, even as this lack of understanding is due to circumstances out of our control.

Some reflection questions here for you to consider:

- Do you have a connection with your ancestors or cultural roots? What does that connection look like? If there is a disconnect, why might that be?

- Which plants are culturally found in your family traditions, whether for food, medicine, decoration, spiritual practices, et cetera?
- What have animals and plants taught you? What can you learn from their guidance?
- Name one thing that produces a feeling of awe or wonder in you. How does that elevate your consciousness?
- Who or what do you have faith in?
- Do you have any daily rituals that help you slow down, be present, and find pleasure in your life?
- Imagine you are free. Free to do anything and be anything. What are you doing? Who are you with? Where are you?

I want to offer you encouragement and love here, my fellow being on this path of reclaiming ancestral practices. Even small steps to being reconnected to your roots are huge and worthwhile.

14

FINDING THE WAY FORWARD

AS I LOOK out into the world, I am reminded that we are in the state of Kali Yuga—the age of darkness where moral virtues and mental capacities are said to be at their lowest. It can feel like an impossible task to look out into the depth of suffering, wondering how to make a difference, but we cannot be lulled into despair. As James Baldwin shared, "Not everything that is faced can be changed, but nothing can be changed until it is faced." I turn to the last line of the Ardās (Sikh prayer) here:

Nanak Naam Chardi Kala, teraa bhane sarbat da bhala.

Oh Nanak, with the name of God comes Chardi Kala and with your blessings comes the well-being for all creation. Chardi Kala is a symbol of hope, resilience, and optimism, and it reminds us that even in the face of adversity, we can always move forward and make progress. Sarbat da bhala means "the well-being of all," and teaches that we should always strive to act in a way that benefits all humanity. This includes being compassionate and working to create a more just and equitable world for all. This prayer says that even through adversity, I commit to being on the spiritual path for not only my well-being but for the well-being of humanity. It is a call to anchor into hope. I am heartened by those striving to make the world a better place for all beings—thank you to the activists, artists, poets, student protesters, spiritual practitioners, and others working for collective liberation.

I truly believe that folks are receiving the call to awaken in different ways. Humanity needs each one of us to show up however and in whatever capacity that we can. We all have our individual skills, gifts, and energy to offer. Liberation work requires solidarity, courage, a willingness to see and speak the truth, and *a commitment to see all people and this planet be free and well.* There are varying levels of consciousness among people, so wherever you are in this fight and solidarity for justice and humanity is welcome. *Don't doubt what you can offer, my love—and how you begin.* We have baby activists and those getting into civic engagement for the first time. We have elders who have been doing this liberation work for lifetime(s). We have those who have lost relationships, aren't speaking to their family members, or feel deeply betrayed and hurt. Some are using their immense grief and anger to channel a better world for all beings. Others are having tough conversations with the people nearest and dearest to them. We have truth tellers on the ground, sharing to social media, and doing critical analysis. We have action takers—those organizing, going to protests, boycotting, disrupting spaces, and planning direct actions. Some folks are using their financial privilege and donating. Others are doing spirit and land work, holding spaces to grieve and process, creating art, and educating. We have those who don't know what to do or how to help. And some deliberately create more hatred, violence, and division.

This is the time to come together and build solidarity. To know we are not alone in this horrific witnessing of genocide, apartheid, greed, occupation, and slavery. We need community to co-regulate and to process this unthinkable amount of violence and trauma occurring. *We cannot do it alone—it is simply not possible.* So, wherever you are, my love, begin the work or continue the good work. This upheaval of oppressive forces and systems is going to take so many of us, coming at it from different ways. We are a part of a building of a new world where there is enough for everybody. Where love, care, and abundance overflow. *Whatever action, small or large, keep going. We cannot be lulled back into complacency.*

Where there is despair, *may we plant seeds of regenerative hope.* Where there is unthinkable violence, *may we learn to stand with and for justice and humanity*. May we tap into our own power to know that we can all make a difference. May we plant as many seeds of love, interconnection, courage, and strength as we can. *May all beings be free.* May Palestinians, Congolese, Sudanese, and all oppressed peoples be free. May the oppressors know their humanity will return when they learn to see all beings as themselves.

I arrive to the conclusion of this book with a call for us to make an effort. Composing this book has been my contribution to doing just that. Having been raised with Sikhism, I have been taught that to be a spiritual practitioner means caring about the suffering of others. So even when the task feels impossible—the task of reclaiming and sharing our ancestral practices with integrity, and the task of alleviating suffering—we don't give up. It does not matter if you have mastered all the poses, know every single pranayama technique, or can sit for hours in meditation *if you are not trying to live ethically*. True spiritual practice is about the acknowledgment of our interconnectedness and our sincere efforts to make a positive difference. It means acknowledging that if I hurt you, other beings, or the land, I am hurting myself. It is acknowledging that we all make up an ecosystem where we are intricately connected. We might not see great changes in our lifetimes, but that does not mean we do not try.

However, not all yogic and spiritual communities orient themselves to this approach. I came out of a five-day Vedic storytelling retreat where the all-white teacher team spoke about spiritual teachings without putting them into context in what is going on in our modern world. In this space, there were about five folks of color and forty-five white folks. I think it is important to learn about these stories from the Mahabharata, the Ramayana, Bhagavad Gita, and Bhagavat Purana to learn the Indian classical stories; however, even within these stories run layers of caste, power over dynamics, and patriarchy. We need to be able to contextualize and tap into the nuances with what is known as *revisionist myth making*. It is not enough to learn about these myths and stories; we must understand how caste, patriarchy, and classism are embedded into these myths. Otherwise, we normalize these -isms and continue to perpetuate a phallocentric cultural system. As Indian author Beena G. comments in her book *Vision and Re-vision: Revisiting Mythology, Rethinking Women*, "Revisionist myth making counters hegemonic narratives and is commonly used as a strategy by writers with an objective of revaluing the experiences of the marginalized people." By reexamining the past through a fresh lens, people who have been historically marginalized can challenge long-held assumptions and gain a deeper understanding of themselves. This process is essential for breaking free from the destructive patterns of an oppressive society.

If we turn to the margas of yoga, we can use those as a remainder to orient ourselves to our interconnectedness and dedication to collective liberation. Jnana yoga is the realization of our true nature and the knowledge that we are all interconnected. Bhakti yoga is recognizing that we are all divine, seeing all beings as divine, and treating them with love. Raja yoga is learning how to control the senses, desires, and impulses to minimize our negative impact on the world. Karma yoga is using the resources we have to act in the service of others without any attachment to the fruit of the action.

What kind of world do you want to live in? What kind of future do you want to see? Right after attending the Vedic storytelling retreat, I went to Deer Park Monastery for their BIPOC retreat and was affirmed that the way forward is going to be led by QTBIPOC, and the way that we are going to get free is through decolonization.

Authentically Engaging with Yoga

Yoga is a sacred practice that should be practiced with respect and reverence. It is a body of knowledge, philosophy, practices, and path that lays out how to approach life, how to meet it, and how to live it with a deeper understanding and appreciation. T. K. V. Desikachar reminds us of this in his translation of Yoga Sutra 2.1 in his book *The Heart of Yoga*: "The practice of Yoga must reduce both physical and mental impurities. It must develop our capacity for self-examination and help us understand that, in the final analysis, we are not the masters of everything that we do."

We are studying these Eastern subjects with a Western lens which impacts how we learn. So how can people practice with more respect? Simply put, by acknowledging where yoga comes from. Here are a couple of ways to do that:

Create your own roots of yoga and spiritual lineage acknowledgment and have this be something you regularly reflect on and refer to. Place this acknowledgment on your website, in your teaching space, and in other places where people would be able to see it. Here is an example of mine:

> *I pay gratitude to all the teachers and practitioners before me, who have kept these teachings alive through centuries of colonization, oppression, patriarchy, empire, and racism. I acknowledge and honor yoga as a spiritual practice originating from the people of South Asia and strive to also keep these teachings alive with humility and reverence. I commit to applying these teachings for the greater good of humanity and to uplift all beings and the earth. I vow to practice inclusion and to bring these practices to where they are needed most.*
>
> *I bow deeply to my teachers, ancestors, to the moon, sun, sky, stars, and to the elements that make up all life. I honor the nature of interconnectedness and acknowledge that without them, I would not be here.*
>
> *May the merits of this practice benefit all beings.*

I encourage you to sit in self-reflection and come up with your own statement. Something that reflects your values and pays homage to where yoga comes from. I also suggest listing out each of your teachers. Having this for myself helped make both my practice and teaching much more meaningful and intentional. Acknowledging your teachers, whether on a website or in person, is a meaningful way to honor their influence on your life, practice, and teachings. Every time I have the privilege of guiding a prenatal yoga student, I express my deep gratitude to Juliana Mitchell. Her years of dedicated practice, embodied knowledge, and the prenatal training she imparted to me has made it possible for me to share this transformative practice with others. Without her wisdom, compassion, and generosity, I wouldn't be able to do what I do today.

This idea is similar to Indigenous land acknowledgments, which I also encourage students and folks to have and use. An example of one I personally use is:

> *We recognize that we are on the unceded ancestral lands of the Tongva, Tataviam, Serrano, Kizh, and Chumash Peoples, who have lived in, cared for, and maintained a deep connection to this land, now colonially known as Los Angeles. I ask you to join me in honoring and respecting their elders—past, present, and emerging—and acknowledge that the legacies of settler colonialism have caused land theft, displacement, broken promises, and lasting trauma. This acknowledgment represents our commitment to truth, healing, and reconciliation and to supporting the stories, cultures, and rights of the original stewards of this land. We are grateful for the privilege to live and work here and pledge to build and sustain respectful, meaningful relationships with Native communities and tribal governments.*

It is important to note here that this is the beginning of the process of reflection, repair, and reparations, not just a box to check. We must create relationships with living Indigenous peoples and learn from them. In undoing settler colonialism, we also acknowledge that many of us are inhabiting lands that are not our own and have been stolen through violence. The Land Back movement calls for the reclamation of everything stolen from Indigenous peoples—land, language, ceremony, housing, governance, and more. Organizers of this movement wish to rebuild symbiotic relationships with the land to stop the exploitation and pollution, revitalize Indigenous ways of life, and be given governance and leadership back over the lands. I believe it is our responsibility as non-Indigenous folks to help repair this harm and turn to Indigenous organizers and movement leaders for guidance. The NDN Collective headed by Nick Tilsen is a great organization to learn from, support, and give back to.

Study yoga's history and the history of South Asia and encourage your local studios to include this important knowledge in their yoga teacher trainings. A lot of trainings spend 70 to 95 percent of their time focused on asana poses, sequencing, and anatomy, which is very important but is not the full picture. In this study of yoga's history, it is also important to reflect on integral work like anti-racism and anti-oppression because, as we covered in this book, even yoga's own histories includes its own legacies of harm. Who we learn from also matters—not all South Asians are a monolith but come from different backgrounds of experience, privilege, and upbringing. The term *pluriversal futures* refers to a vision or possibility of the future that recognizes and honors the coexistence of diverse views, cultures, and ways of being. Diversify the South Asian and QTBIPOC teachers whom you are learning from. Stay open and respectful and listen to varying members of the source culture when they teach you about their heritage, traditions, lineage, and practices. As Chimamanda Ngozi Adiche said, "The danger of a single story is that it robs people of their dignity."

Who you learn from colors your perspective on history. Ever heard of the phrase "History is written by the victors"? I go further here and say the "victors" are typically those who have colonized, murdered, stolen, and written history to paint themselves in a better light. I think about learning *real* US history after going through years of brainwashing and realizing what a villain the US is. This is why it is important to learn from a diverse group of people, especially those from oppressed backgrounds—we get a different viewpoint of history that paints a truer picture. Commit to amplifying and learning from QTBIPOC who have been historically marginalized and erased in wellness and healing culture.

When it comes to learning and studying yoga, having community, a good teacher, and guidance is important. A yoga student doesn't need to, and really shouldn't, pursue this study in isolation. Find a teacher, community, and space that aligns with you. Discern and then commit. I teach online as a part of the Tejal Yoga community, and I have found this to be a supportive and healing place. Tejal Yoga is a South Asian, teacher-led yoga community focused on educating and empowering every yoga student in the world about social justice and decolonizing wellness actions.

Studentship is most important—keep studying and living your yoga. To be a student of yoga is to be a student of life. Yoga is not meant to be learned and integrated in a 200-hour training. It is a lifetime(s) path of self-inquiry, study, and practice, and it is a path and practice that is meant to be lived. Yoga is not about information collection; it is about wisdom gleaned and applied.

Doing one or even multiple trainings does not make you a master in someone else's culture. To carry the lineage of another culture entails establishing and nurturing a deep, enduring relationship with the culture and its people. Cultural humility is important. And don't compare your journey to someone else's. This rush to be at the same level or better is a symptom of capitalism. Give yourself the grace to go at your own pace and growth level.

This is where your personal sadhana (sincere and dedicated spiritual practice) comes in. It is vital as yoga students and teachers to maintain a personal practice—whether it is pranayama, prayer, meditation, seva, reading of wisdom texts, asana, or something else. Through a committed practice with abhyasa (continuous practice) and vairagya (consistent letting go), we create intentional time and space to connect with ourselves and deepen our self-knowledge. It creates a container to tune into oneself. I encourage students to practice at least five times a week, if even for only five minutes, and slowly start to extend that awareness and grace into every aspect of your life. A sadhana is personal, and only the practitioner and a trusted teacher is able to reflect on how it is impacting them.

Know when to say you don't know and admit when you are wrong. There is no shame in not knowing something. In school, we get bad grades for not knowing something, and that teaches us that if we don't know, we are stupid or bad. However, in yoga, there is an understanding that avidya (ignorance) is something innate to all human beings. We can't learn something without first realizing we don't know it. Be malleable and understand that you will never know everything and that your practice can be subject to change. Admit that there is always more learning and growth to be had; reach for that wisdom.

Especially as a teacher, make sure you have practiced something before you teach it. For example, if you don't practice meditation and haven't studied it, then don't teach it. Bring the reverence and devotion back to these practices. We are always yoga students before we are yoga professionals or teachers. Be patient. And work with satya (truthfulness). Let your students know if you don't know something—something like "I don't have the answer to that" or "I will strive to get back to you or recommend another person or resource." I find this creates trust because we are dropping the mask of needing to know it all and be perfect.

Take the time and intention to connect to your own ancestors and cultural lineage and have your own ancestral practices. This is a call to be in right relationship with other cultures through looking at, processing, and integrating your own cultural wounds and ancestral trauma. This is a challenge to white folks to understand their own ancestral lineages and see what practices they hold. To stop taking from other cultures. And this is a call for you to learn about your own history and connect to your culture, whatever that might be. This can be complex work that can bring with it grief, confusion, anger, and other feelings, so be gentle with yourself.

Yoga brought me closer and deeper to myself and my culture and back to Sikhism. I found a sense of belonging *and* it forced me to see the legacies of internalized colonialism, colorism, interreligious conflict, and harm that has also been caused by and to my ancestors. Being in right relationship means admitting when our ancestral lineage has caused harm and working to repair that. For white folks, that might bring up a lot, and it is worthwhile work because the appropriation, exploitation, and harm is still occurring all over the world.

Learn from, hire, and uplift South Asian and BIPOC yoga teachers. Give more than just credit and involve the original stewards of this practice in the conversation. We shouldn't be marginalized and invisible in our ancestral and cultural practices. White folks, use your power, privilege, and money to give back to South Asian and BIPOC teachers. If you are part of a studio, yoga organization, festival, or conference and notice there isn't any South Asian or BIPOC representation, consider it your responsibility to say something and invite these teachers in. We need you as a supporter and ally. Speak up, highlight the inequities, and hold yourself and others accountable. Don't be complicit in systems and organizations that exploit, appropriate, and commodify yoga and the culture. This is cultural violence.

And for South Asian and BIPOC folks, don't fall into the trap of tokenism, alignment with white supremacy, and competition. Tokenism assumes that one or a few people can speak up for an entire group of people. Going beyond this looks like inviting more diverse voices. There is room for more than just one BIPOC in these spaces. Uplift others alongside you. The British colonial rulers used a divide and conquer strategy in India during their period of colonialism. The strategy aimed to maintain control and dominance by fostering divisions and conflicts among the South Asian population. We shouldn't play into this legacy of colonialism by being divided among ourselves.

Move past self-care to community care. Many of us turned to yoga because of the physical, mental, emotional, and spiritual relief and ease it brought into our life. And then many of those people became teachers to extend that same medicine to others—there is a deep sense of purpose there. Yoga has been life-giving because when I teach it, I am receiving something just as much as I am giving it. In a retreat I attended, Dr. Robert Svoboda shared that yoga teachers and doctors have the most karma associated with their professions—so practice with integrity.

Pathway to Liberation

A wise person can hold different complexities and multiple truths. I want to hold and honor the transformative power of the practices we have today while also holding and recognizing the oppression that is flowing through these practices. This is part of the messiness of life. None of this is black and white. I do not wish to devalue someone's asana practice if it has transformed their life, as it also has done for me—and at the same time, I do want to look at how asana has been stripped out and pulled out of context.

A big way of moving forward is to deconstruct and dissolve ego identities that hold us from understanding ourselves and developing ethical virtues. It is to integrate ethical virtues and personal values and put them into action.

Why are you practicing yoga? Why are you teaching it?

We can begin decolonizing our practice by looking at the original intents and goals of yoga and implementing those in our life. These are self-realization, freedom, interconnectedness, and service.

What does it look like to recenter these holistic and inclusive goals in your own practice? How does the nature of your practice start to change?

Anyone who calls themselves a yoga teacher or a yoga student must honestly ask themselves if their yoga practice is truly making them a self-inquiring person who stays accountable to and cares for their community. We all have a role to play in creating impactful change in our communities. Yoga can be used as a tool of liberatory change, and I encourage all of us to tap into the full power and potential of the path and the practice.

As yoga expands in popularity, I imagine we will see more trends pop up within the space. We have nude yoga, punk yoga, goat yoga, hot yoga, power yoga, and I'm sure we will have the next big craze + yoga soon. Is there a way to stop this? I don't think there is, but I do think there is more space for students, practitioners, and teachers who want to understand the whole of yoga to understand themselves, to grow, and then expand their wisdom and capacity to help others. To those folks: We need your heart guided and service focused approach. Please know that the world needs you. Keep learning and flourishing on this path. Trends will come and go, but a commitment to the heart qualities of yoga will remain with the sincere students.

T. K. V. Desikachar said his father Krishnamacharya had more notes and things to say about the Yoga Sutras over the years. Every time he studied it and he combined with his own life experience, he understood something new on a deeper level. I love this because it teaches us that we will always be learning and realizing on this path. Life experience is key in yoga. There will always be more to know and realize. Even from the same text! It is a good practice to come back and keep revisiting.

Thich Nhat Hanh said the next Buddha will be the sangha, and I agree with this. I see the future as flourishing yoga communities where people see and hear one another, learn, and grow. Where people of various identities are included and celebrated. It is a lifelong commitment. I see spaces where there is a deep commitment to studentship, humility, and striving to apply the teachings to make conditions better for all beings. Community helps to keep each other accountable.

It's often said that the more we think we know and understand, the more we realize there is so much that we don't know and may never know or understand. I've come to realize this as I've continued to walk my own path, and especially as I've worked on this book, gathering insights from others and mining my own experiences for wisdom. There is infinite depth and scope for how we continue in the face of what we know and don't know in terms of yoga and our lives. We have the tools, the teachings, and the wisdom that lie within us and among us and on which we can call. I hope that what I have shared with you has resonated on some level, and if it has, the credit must go to my teachers. Any inaccuracies are my mistake in interpretation alone. This is how I accept accountability and strive to move with integrity. I encourage and wish for you to do the same. May we connect to the wisdom and compassion within our hearts, to the truth of our interconnectedness and our interdependence to all beings, and to the strength and resilience of our spirits. We are in relation with everything around us—the plants, lands, bugs, birds, humans, the skies. I pray we learn to listen more deeply and love everything as a part of us, because it is. May we all find our individual and collective way forward toward total liberation.

ACKNOWLEDGMENTS

This book would not have been possible without the support of those around me, the collective experiences of my students, and the deeply personal journey that has shaped my understanding of yoga. I am forever grateful to the following individuals:

To my beloved partner of ten years, Dr. Ali Esmaeili—you are the unwavering foundation beneath my feet. You are the embodiment of Buddha-nature itself, radiating compassion, empathy, generosity, and wisdom for all beings. I practice to be more like you. Thank you for being my sounding board and steadfast support throughout the writing of this book. I love you deeply.

To my in-laws, Asghar Esmaeili, who immigrated from Iran to the United States, and Merlyn Esmaeili, who came from the Philippines, thank you for creating a nurturing space for me to write and providing the resources and environment I needed to do so in peace. You have shown me the true meaning of belonging and being part of a family that is steady, regulated, and full of love. I am especially grateful for our nightly chats around the dinner table, where we discussed resistance fighters across the globe, the dangers of imperialism and empire, and envisioned a world beyond a US-centered perspective.

To Tia Brandt, my best friend of twelve years—thank you for being my cheerleader and for always encouraging me to pursue my dreams. I still remember that day we were kayaking at Bonelli Lake, contemplating whether I should write this book. Your gentle nudges and heartfelt belief in me helped spark the courage I needed to take this leap. You are not only my favorite person in the world, but also my partner for life, and I am so grateful for the countless memories we've created together. Here's to many more adventures and dreams realized side by side!

To my parents, Paramjit Kaur and Mann Singh, I am grateful for your devotion to Sikhism and for raising me in its rich traditions. As an adult, I've grown more of an appreciation, through my own seeking and understanding. To my grandmother, Amar Kaur (Bibiji), thank you for instilling in me a fire for justice and a strong sense of right and wrong through your no-nonsense attitude.

To all my teachers: This book is a testament to your wisdom and guidance. Deepest of gratitude to Paramhansa Yogananda, Nayaswami Narayan, Juliana Mitchell, Charlotte Nguyen, T. K. V. Desikachar, Siri Bahadur Khalsa, Mehtab Benton, Steph "Navjeet" Smith, Miriam Van Doorn, Thich Nhat Hanh, Sister Dang Ngheim, Guru Nanak, Durga Mata, Zabie Yamasaki, Kaya Mindlin, Dr. Scott Blossom, S. N. Goenka, and Dr. Miles Neale. Your teachings continue to shape my path. Without y'all, this book would not be.

A special thank you goes to my teacher and mentor, Sri Prasad Rangnekar, who guided me through moments of self-doubt and confusion, held me accountable, and offered firm support and encouragement. In our conversations, your directness consistently cut to the heart of the matter—a clarity I needed and cherish. You are a true lighthouse of wisdom, illuminating the path for so many, myself included. I bow deeply to you, dear teacher.

To all those who generously offered their time through interviews and answering my questions: Susanna Barkataki, Kendra Coupland, Dr. Neil Dalal, Reggie Hubbard, Tejal Patel, Anjali Rao, Dr. Shyam Ranganathan, Leah Saliter, and Channdika Valli. Your insights and perspectives were invaluable.

To my assistant, Sabrina Joan Hughes—thank you for being the first to read my manuscript and for providing invaluable feedback that fueled me to keep going. Your humor and loyal support have been a constant light, making this journey, and my life, so much easier.

To Joelle Hann and Aliya Mughal, my incredible book coaches and editors, you held my hand through the fog of uncertainty and lifted me from moments of hesitation. Thank you for being my compass when I felt lost and for helping me see this project through to completion. You both helped create a scaffolding for this book to take form—thank you.

To Andrew DeYoung and the team at Broadleaf Books: This book would not exist without Andrew's initial outreach. Your belief in this project and your steady hand helped fortify my vision. Thank you for our calls where you played the roles of both publisher and therapist, if you ever decide to switch careers, you have a calling! To the extraordinary team at Broadleaf Books, especially my editors, Erin Gibbons, Marissa Uhrina, and Hannah Varacalli, thank you for your support and guidance in turning my messy manuscript into an actual book.

To Hope Glastris, Meera Dhawan, and Kiran Vajapey, my heartfelt thanks for bringing this book's cover to life. The symbolism of Anjali mudra holds profound significance—it embodies the unity of mind and heart, serves as a gesture of respect, and reflects the healing journey this book aims to inspire. Anjali mudra signifies the potential for intention to evolve into spiritual awakening. When executed properly, the palms are not flat against one another; instead, the knuckles at the base of the fingers bend slightly, creating a space that resembles a flower yet to bloom, symbolizing the potential for the opening of our hearts. Spiritual growth is possible for each and every single one of us.

To Tristan Katz and Melissa Shah, thank you for taking the time to read the manuscript and shedding light on areas where I needed to acknowledge my privilege and strive for greater awareness. Your insights have been instrumental in deepening the impact of this work.

I want to express my heartfelt gratitude to the Glendora Public Library and the Sanctuary Cafe for being the spaces where I accomplished much of my writing. These environments were not just locations; they were sources of inspiration and solace. Libraries, in particular, have always held a special place in my heart. Books gave me the world, showing me characters who lived in alternate ways and modeled ways to overcome struggle and strife. It was through books that I found my sense of belonging and purpose, and I cannot overstate how much the stories I encountered have shaped who I am today. It's essential to continue providing funding for libraries, as they open doors to countless possibilities for others.

To all my students—thank you. Without you, I would not be a teacher. You continue to teach me as much as I teach you. This book is for you. Especially to those in the Tejal Yoga Sangha, I have been guiding this community and teaching most of these students for the last three-plus years every Monday morning at 7:00. Y'all's dedication inspires me and warms my heart! My students' care, wisdom, and vulnerability continue to encourage me to be better every day. Your curious questions centered around the why propel me to go deeper into yoga. To the teens I've worked with and continue to work with, I want a more safe and kind world for you.

To my healed ancestors and spirit guides: I feel your presence and support, seen and unseen. Your strength flows through me. Thank you for loving me and for your protection and blessings.

To the lands of South Asia and India: I honor these sacred lands, where yoga was born and has been preserved for centuries, even through colonialism, violence, appropriation, and land theft. I am grateful to the teachers who retreated into caves, forests, and monasteries to gain insights into the nature of reality and who kept these teachings alive for future generations. We are indebted to the yogis of the past for their studies and acquired wisdom, so now we can turn to this ancient and innate wisdom to guide our paths.

To yoga: Words are not enough to express my gratitude. This path has saved my life and given me meaning. My love for yoga is boundless and it continues to be my source of healing, freedom, and liberation.

Finally, to all who have walked this journey with me—your support, seen and unseen, has lifted me every step of the way. I am profoundly grateful for each person, each lesson, and each moment of grace that has brought this book into being. From the bottom of my heart, thank you.

NOTES

Introduction: The Journey to Wholeness

2. ***This brokenness is evidenced:*** Sally C. Curtin and Matthew F. Garnett, "Suicide and Homicide Death Rates among Youth and Young Adults Aged 10–24: United States, 2001–2021", no. 471 (2023).

Chapter 1: My Search for Belonging

8. ***keep it covered as protection:*** Bhai Randheer Singh Ji, *Anhad Shabad Dasam Duar*, accessed November 10, 2023, https://www.vidhia.com/Bhai%20Randheer%20Singh%20Ji/Anhad-shabad-dasam-duar.pdf.
15. ***higher risk of poor mental health:*** Fiza Pirani, "Issue 08: What If No Place Feels Like Home?", Foreign Bodies (blog), July 31, 2019, https://foreignbodies.substack.com/p/when-no-place-feels-like-home-19-08-01.

Chapter 2: Reconnecting to Yoga's Roots

27. ***we will get only temporary states of peace:*** Miles Neale, "On McMindfulness and Frozen Yoga: Rediscovering the Essential Teachings of Ethics and Wisdom," InsightTimer (blog), 2011, https://insighttimer.com/blog/mcmindfulness-frozen-yoga-miles-neale/.
28. ***"The root of affliction is past action":*** Patanjali's Yoga Sūtra, trans. Shyam Ranganathan (New York: Penguin Classics, 2008), 148.
29. ***we are losing the deeper spiritual:*** Neale, "On McMindfulness and Frozen Yoga."
34. ***the experience of an individual soul:*** Suzanne Newcombe, "The Revival of Yoga in Contemporary India," in *Oxford Research Encyclopedia of Religion* (Oxford University Press, 2017), 10.1093/acrefore/9780199340378.013.253.

Chapter 3: Asana as Freedom from Physical Fixation

39. ***asana is mentioned in only three of the 196 total sutras:*** Ranganathan, Patanjali's Yoga Sūtra.
41. ***Yoga Journal has been criticized:*** Sana Saeed, Sarah Nasr, and Kathryn Wheeler, "Why Americans Are So Obsessed with Yoga," AJ+, March 25, 2018, https://www.youtube.com/watch?v=lSkxAh8QT-o.
41. ***In these earlier issues:*** Nyk Danu, "Why I Boycott Yoga Journal (and Think You Should Too)," *Elephant Journal*, August 26, 2020, https://www.elephantjournal.com/2020/07/why-i-boycott-yoga-journal-and-think-you-should-too-nyk-danu/.
42. ***"Racism is so implicit":*** Amy Champ, "Why Your Yoga Class Is So White," interview by Rosalie Murphy, *The Atlantic*, July 8, 2014. https://www.theatlantic.com/national/archive/2014/07/why-your-yoga-class-is-so-white/374002/.
43. ***"The algorithm favors certain qualities":*** Sakshi Venkatraman, "White Women Co-Opted Pandemic Yoga. Now, South Asian Instructors Are Taking It Back," *NBC News*, April 13, 2021, https://www.nbcnews.com/news/asian-america/white-women-co-opted-pandemic-yoga-now-south-asian-instructors-n1263952.
52. ***"My father never saw":*** T. K. V. Desikachar, *The Heart of Yoga: Developing a Personal Practice* (Rochester, VT: Inner Traditions International, 1999).
53. ***"To the yogi":*** Andrea R. Jain, *Selling Yoga: From Counterculture to Pop Culture*, 1st ed (Oxford University Press, 2013), 82.
53. ***"instruction is confined":*** Suzanne Newcombe, "The Institutionalization of the Yoga Tradition: 'Gurus' B. K. S. Iyengar and Yogini Sunita in Britain," in *Gurus of Modern Yoga*, ed. Mark Singleton and Ellen Goldberg (New York: Oxford University Press), 147–167.
56. ***"Ignorance is the notion":*** Ranganathan, Patanjali's Yoga Sūtra.
57. ***"It cannot be overstated":*** Edwin Bryant, *The Yoga Sutras of Patañjali: A New Edition, Translation, and Commentary* (New York: North Point Press, 2015), xl.

Chapter 4: The Many Paths (Margas) of Yoga

61. ***The poem "A Great Yogi":*** Jerry Zehr, "Centering," in *The Peacemaker's Path: Multifaith Reflections to Deepen Your Spirituality*, (Minneapolis, MN: Broadleaf Books, 2021), 40.
66. ***"The means to liberation":*** Ranganathan, Patanjali's Yoga Sūtra.

Chapter 5: How The Trauma of Colonialism Lives in Our Bones

79. ***"And it wasn't long before":*** "What Is CorePower Yoga? About Us & Our Mission," CorePower Yoga, https://www.corepoweryoga.com/content/about-us.
80. ***By the mid-twentieth century:*** Jason Hickel, "How Britain Stole $45 Trillion from India," *Al Jazeera*, December 19, 2018, https://www.aljazeera.com/opinions/2018/12/19/how-britain-stole-45-trillion-from-india.
81. ***Over the next several decades:*** Shashi Tharoor, *An Era of Darkness. The British Empire in India* (New Delhi: Aleph, 2016).
81. ***They deliberately sowed seeds:*** Tharoor, *An Era of Darkness.*
82. ***"Whites did not simply gain":*** Steve Martinot, "The Dual-State Character of U.S. Coloniality: Notes toward Decolonization," *Human Architecture: Journal of the Sociology of Self-Knowledge* V (2007): 371–82, https://www.okcir.com/product/journal-article-the-dual-state-character-of-u-s-coloniality-notes-toward-decolonization-by-steve-martinot/.
83. ***The British showed little concern:*** Shashi Tharoor, "The Partition: The British Game of 'Divide and Rule,'" *Al Jazeera*, August 10, 2017, https://www.aljazeera.com/opinions/2017/8/10/the-partition-the-british-game-of-divide-and-rule.
84. ***"When British rule in India":*** Amara Miller, "The Origins of Yoga: Part III," The Sociological Yogi (blog), September 23, 2014, https://amaramillerblog.wordpress.com/2014/05/29/the-origins-of-yoga-part-iii/.
85. ***"not only inferior but parasitic":*** Miller, "The Origins of Yoga."
86. ***"And so, people start creating":*** Dr. Shyam Ranganathan (researcher and scholar), in discussion with author, Zoom,

April 2023. Transcript available on www.harpindermann.com.

87. ***"To many Hindus":*** "The Third Gender and Hijras," ed. Diane L. Moore (Harvard Divinity School, 2018), https://hwpi.harvard.edu/files/rpl/files/gender_hinduism.pdf?m=1597338930.
90. ***"It is a radical act to breathe":*** Michelle Cassandra Johnson, *Skill in Action: Radicalizing Your Yoga Practice to Create a Just World* (Boulder, CO: Shambhala Publications, 2021).

Chapter 6: Unpacking Our Role in the Decolonization Journey

94. ***"getting to the fundamental root":*** Mojdeh Cox, "Mojdeh Cox on the Anatomy of Radical Accountability," Pillar Nonprofit Network, https://pillarnonprofit.ca/news/mojdeh-cox-anatomy-radical-accountability.
96. ***During Buddha's period:*** James Mallinson and Mark Singleton, *Roots of Yoga* (London: Penguin, 2017), 51.
98. ***Yoga was practiced and studied:*** "History of Yoga," Vishuddhi Films, April 1, 2022, https://www.youtube.com/watch?v=JoRwXMLsVis.
99. ***Some argue this is evidence:*** Yan Y. Dhyansky, "The Indus Valley Origin of a Yoga Practice," *Artibus Asiae* 48, no. 1/2 (1987): 89–108, https://doi.org/10.2307/3249853. Georg Feuerstein, *The Yoga Tradition: Its History, Literature, Philosophy and Practice* (Prescott, AZ: Hohm Press, 1998), 100.
99. ***Carvings show people:*** Dianne Bondy, "The Black History of Yoga: A Short Exploration of Kemetic Yoga," Home, February 5, 2021, https://yogainternational.com/article/view/the-black-history-of-yoga/.
99. ***It is believed that the Aryans:*** The early Iranians self-identified as Aryan, meaning "noble" or "free," and the term continued in use for over two thousand years until it was corrupted by European racists to serve their own agenda (https://www.worldhistory.org/Indus_Valley_Civilization/).
101. ***Preserved through Sramanic traditions:*** Thenmozhi Soundararajan, *The Trauma of Caste: A Dalit Feminist Meditation on*

Survivorship, Healing, and Abolition (Oakland, CA: North Atlantic Books, 2022), 66. Govind Chandra Pande, *Studies in the Origins of Buddhism* (Allahabad: Department of Ancient History, Culture, and Archeology, Unibersitu of Allahabad, 1957), 251–309.

102. ***"There was a plurality":*** Edwin Bryant, *The Yoga Sutras of Patañjali: A New Edition, Translation, and Commentary* (New York: North Point Press, 2015).
102. ***From 600 to 1300 CE:*** Remember from chapter 4 that religion did not exist in South Asia during this time as we understand it now. What existed were varying philosophical traditions and ways of being and connecting to the divine. And there were many different traditions; even Hinduism as we understand it now has different denominations underneath it.
102. ***This period is important:*** Goodall, Dominic, "Śaiva Tantra: Toward a History," in *The Oxford Handbook of Tantric Studies*, ed. Richard K. Payne and Glen A. Hayes (online ed., Oxford Academic, 18 Aug. 2022), https://doi.org/10.1093/oxfordhb/9780197549889.013.45.
104. ***"does not mean a shift":*** Sheena Sood, "Towards a Critical Embodiment of Decolonizing Yoga," *Race and Yoga* 5, no. 1 (2020): 7, https://doi.org/10.5070/r351049160.
104. ***I understand it to be a long-term process:*** Sood, "Towards a Critical Embodiment."

Chapter 7: Yoga Mats, Yoga Pants, and Expensive Classes

112. ***I found a product review:*** Jia Tolentino, "These $108 Lululemon Meditation Beads Seem Worth It," *Jezebel*, January 12, 2015, https://jezebel.com/these-108-lululemon-meditation-beads-seem-worth-it-1678958675.
114. ***In the traditional writings:*** Ranganathan, Patanjali's Yoga Sūtra.
115. ***It is in the critique:*** Bryant, *The Yoga Sutras*.
118. ***"Consider New Age logic":*** bell hooks, *All About Love: New Visions* (New York: William Morrow, 1999).
120. ***We keep running:*** Bryant, *The Yoga Sutras*.

Chapter 8: The Nuances of Appropriation and Practicing with Integrity

128. ***Additionally, the historical:*** "Racism Defined," DRWorksBook, May 2021, https://www.dismantlingracism.org/racism-defined.html.
129. ***Capitalism has led to globalization:*** Sourabh Yadav and Chris Drew, "Dominant Culture: Definition and 10 Examples," *Helpful Professor*, September 6, 2023, https://helpfulprofessor.com/dominant-culture/.
129. ***Power Over is the power:*** "Power," JASS, accessed October 28, 2023, https://justassociates.org/what-we-do/power/.
129. ***In his groundbreaking 1978 book:*** Edward W. Said, *Orientalism* (London: Routledge & Kegan Paul, 1978).
130. ***"The thing about cultural appropriation":*** Sonny Singh Brooklynwala, "Turbans on the Runway," *The Langar Hall*, July 10, 2012, https://thelangarhall.com/entertainment/turbans-on-the-runway-what-does-it-mean-for-sikhs/.
131. ***This hate group came out:*** Ricardo Kaulessar, "How Indians in Jersey City Fought Back against the Terror of 'Dotbusters' in the 1980s," *North Jersey Media Group*, March 29, 2023, https://www.northjersey.com/story/news/new-jersey/2022/01/26/indians-jersey-city-nj-attacks-1980-s/6397092001/.
133. ***"I remember when I started":*** Elisa Lipsky-Karasz, "Gwyneth Paltrow Wants to Convert You," the *Wall Street Journal*, December 4, 2018, https://www.wsj.com/articles/gwyneth-paltrow-wants-to-convert-you-1543931659.
136. ***This means "Get up":*** Indu Arora, *Yoga: Ancient Heritage, Tomorrow's Vision* (Minneapolis, MN: Yog Sadhna, 2019), 79.
140. ***Everyone is free:*** Daniel Simpson, *The Truth of Yoga: A Comprehensive Guide to Yoga's History, Texts, Philosophy, and Practices* (New York: North Point Press, 2021), 199.

Chapter 9: The Erosion of Spiritual and Cultural Foundations

145. ***"What began as a quest":*** Amanda Lucia, "Representation and Whiteness among the 'Spiritual but Not Religious,'" Canopy Forum, November 23, 2020, https://canopyforum.org/

2020/09/24/representation-and-whiteness-among-the-spiritual-but-not-religious/.

148. ***"soul wound":*** Eduardo Duran, Patricia Grant Long, Barbara Ellen Smith, and Talmage Stanley, "From Historical Trauma to Hope and Healing: 2004 Appalachian Studies Association Conference [with Responses]," *Appalachian Journal* 32, no. 2 (2005): 164–80, http://www.jstor.org/stable/40934391.
149. ***For example, the manifesto:*** Kamal Munir, Shahzad Ansari, and Deborah Brown, "From Patañjali to the 'Gospel of Sweat': Yoga's Remarkable Transformation from a Sacred Movement into a Thriving Global Market," *Administrative Science Quarterly* 66, no. 3 (2021): 854–899, https://doi.org/10.1177/0001839221993475.

Chapter 10: Is Two Hundred Hours Enough?

155. ***The credentialing body:*** "About Us," Yoga Alliance, last updated November 24, 2020, https://www.yogaalliance.org/About_Us/Our_History.
156. ***According to some measures***: Abby McCain, "25+ Interesting Yoga Industry Statistics [2023]: Yoga Trends + Revenue," June 20, 2023, https://www.zippia.com/advice/yoga-industry-statistics/.
157. ***"History is being erased everywhere":*** Anjali Rao (President of the board of directors of Accessible Yoga), in discussion with author, Zoom, April 2023. Transcript available on www.harpindermann.com.

Chapter 11: Spiritual Bypassing Won't Save Us

168. ***He defined it as:*** Sara-Mai Conway, "Spiritual Bypassing and How to Avoid It," *Mindworks*, September 16, 2023, https://mindworks.org/blog/spiritual-bypassing-how-to-avoid/.
169. ***bypassing:*** Sara-Mai Conway, "Spiritual Bypassing and How to Avoid It," Mindworks, July 11, 2023, https://mindworks.org/blog/spiritual-bypassing-how-to-avoid/.
171. ***"simply allowing the thing":*** Lama Rod Owens, *Love and Rage: The Path of Liberation through Anger* (Berkeley, CA: North Atlantic Books, 2020), 152–153.
175. ***"If all you see is white":*** Regina Jackson and Saira Rao, *White Women: Everything You Already Know about Your Own Racism and How to Do Better* (New York: Penguin, 2022).

175. ***"come from their culture":*** Susanna Barkataki, in discussion with author, Zoom, May 2023. Transcript available on www.harpindermann.com.

Chapter 12: The Gift That Yoga Gives Us

183. ***At one point, Sibling Dex:*** Becky Chambers, *A Psalm for the Wild-Built* (New York: Tor, 2021).

Chapter 13: Reclaiming Ancestral Connection One Step at a Time

194. ***"Our spiritual life":*** Dang Nghiem, *Flowers in the Dark: Reclaiming Your Power to Heal from Trauma with Mindfulness* (New York: Random House, 2021), 64.
203. ***"culture":*** Āio (aio.thepodcast), "I'm excited about this one 🙌 exploring reindigenisation as opposed to decolonisation with @learnmaoriabroad," August 21, 2023, https://www.instagram.com/p/CwMm1rGMsKo/.
204. ***"The Master's Tools Will Never Dismantle the Master's House":*** Audre Lorde, *Sister Outsider: Essays and Speeches* (Berkeley, CA: Crossing Press, 2007), 110–114.
205. ***"Whenever Black and Brown people":*** Quoted in Terra Incognita, "Indigenous Peoples' Day and the Connection to Palestine," October 10, 2023.